**Love Your Skin, Love Yourself:** *Achieving Beauty, Health, and Vitality from the Inside Out and Outside In*

Published by Sennin Group, LLC

P.O. Box 71

Wanaque, NJ 07465

www.senningroup.com


Edited by Daniella Thoren

Cover photography: John Agnello Photography and Video

Cover and book design: Michelle Fitz, Hat Trick Strategies, Ltd, www.hattrickstrategies.com


ISBN-10: 061585172X

ISBN-13: 978-0615851723

# Dedication

This book is dedicated to anyone who has experienced insecurity, self doubt, lack of confidence, shame, fear, or any other negative emotion due to a skin condition. You are not alone, there is nothing wrong with you, and there is hope for healing—physically, emotionally, and spiritually.

# Contributors (In alphabetical order)

## Christine Arylo

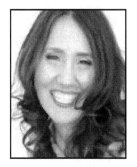

Christine Arylo is a transformational teacher, speaker and best-selling author. After earning her MBA and climbing the corporate ladder, she chose to devote her life to creating a new reality for women and girls, one based on self-love and true feminine power instead of the relentless pursuit of having to do, be and have it all.

She is the author of two best-selling books, *Choosing ME before WE* and *Madly in Love With Me, The Daring Adventure to Becoming Your Own Best Friend*, and the co-founder of *Inner Mean Girl Reform School*, which has helped over 23,000 women transform their inner critics. She is also the founder of the international Day of Self-Love, February 13th. She is affectionately known as 'The Queen of Self-Love.'

Christine has been featured on CBS, ABC, FOX, E!, the Huffington Post, and on radio shows and stages around the world, including TEDx. She normally lives in Northern California with her partner, Noah, but recently they sold their house to live their dream of living, working and speaking and teaching from anywhere in the world. To find out more about Christine go to www.ChristineArylo.com and www.ChooseSelfLove.com

## Dr. Ben Johnson
Osmosis Skincare Founder and Formulator

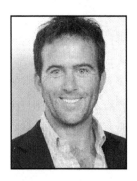

Dr. Ben Johnson started his career in 1997 when he opened one of the first medi-spa chains with locations all around the U.S. Dr. Johnson then founded and formulated his first skin care line, Cosmedix, with a strategy that was unique at the time - creating medical strength results using all natural and chirally correct ingredients.

Dr. Johnson has developed Osmosis Skincare with the goal of changing the direction of skin care away from excessive exfoliation and renewing the focus of dermal remodeling. It works on every skin condition on every skin type. The product range has created a great deal of excitement in the beauty industry, thanks to its unique action and outstanding results. For more information about Dr. Johnson or Osmosis Skincare, please visit www.osmosisskincare.com.

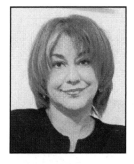

### Sharonah Rapseik
#### Ph.D., ASCP, HHC, AADP

Sharonah Rapseik is the owner of Spa Holistica www.spaholistica.com, a boutique holistic skincare spa located in midtown Manhattan. She is a graduate of the Institute of Integrative Nutrition® and is a certified Dr.Hauschka® Skincare Practitioner.

### Georgia Tetlow
#### MD, FAAPMR

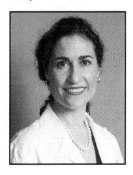

Dr. Tetlow synthesizes the best of conventional and alternative medicine to help individuals regain and maintain health and balance. She holds a faculty affiliation at Thomas Jefferson Medicine College, is board certified in physical medicine and rehabilitation and fellowship trained at the University of Arizona Center for Integrative Medicine. She has expertise in mind-body medicine, biologically-based herbal therapies and diets, and energy medicine to treat chronic illness, cancer recovery and pain. She was certified as a Hatha yoga instructor 20 years ago and encourages all her patients to reap the benefits of a daily mind-body practice. She practices in Ambler, PA, please visit www.philly-im.com, email info@philly-im.com or call (888) 702-7974 to make an appointment.

### Daniella Thoren
#### Editor

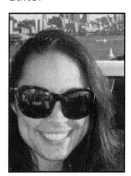

Daniella Thoren graduated from Wagner College in Staten Island, NY, with degrees in English and Journalism. She has spent most of her professional life in the healthcare publishing industry, developing educational content for allied health professionals, advanced practice nurses, and physician assistants and has traveled around the country supporting continuing education at professional conferences. She currently serves as an Associate Publisher with Lippincott, Williams, and Wilkins, Philadelphia.

# Acknowledgements

I've been blessed with wonderful people in my life who have helped me become the person I am today, personally and professionally. Without the guidance, support, and love from the following people, my career would not have its direction and this book might have never been written.

To my husband, Joe Pontillo, for working so hard to support our family as I stayed home with our kids and had the opportunity to go back to school not once but twice to finally figure out what I wanted to be when I grew up! To our girls, Giulia and Giada, for always inspiring me to be a better mother than I was yesterday—I love you all so much.

To my parents and siblings—Cathy, Carmine, Cheryl, Rebecca, Nick—and to Kathy, Bob, and Laura for all the inspiration, love, and support through the years.

To my amazing friend and editor, Daniella Thoren, it's because of you that I ever started writing at all. I've learned so much from working with you over the years and I've cherished our friendship along the way. Thank you for taking this project on, for making my words clearer, and for all of the supportive comments, direction, and constructive criticism. Your work made this book the best it can be. Thank you.

To my friend Manoj Abraham, for inspiring me that I could even write a book at all. Thanks also for all of your advice and support during this process and for your amazing work on my website.

To my friend Tisha Palmer, for all the long talks and brainstorming sessions—for always listening and never judging—for sharing your many gifts. You are a gem.

To my friend and cohort, Alicia Kushmaul—thanks for the amazing creative and logistic support and for being one of my greatest cheerleaders. I'm so happy to have you in my "corner" and can't wait to see what we come up with next!

To my coaches and teachers—Brenda Kress, Joshua Rosenthal, Marie Forleo, Alicia Dunams, and countless others—your out-of-the box thinking, innovation, wisdom, and support have inspired me in so many ways—I am forever grateful.

To Jim Flynn, for all the generous advice and guidance, and for helping me make sure all my bases are covered.

To Sara Iannaccone, thank you for being a last minute fresh set of eyes!

To my clients and readers—Thank you for sharing your stories, your emotions, your struggles, and your triumphs with me. Thank you for trusting me to walk alongside you on your journey. I'm honored to be part of your life and am grateful to be of service.

# Contents

# Introduction

Achieving good and healthy skin has always been important to me because I wasn't blessed with it. I dealt with acne from the time I was a tween all the way into my early thirties. When I was a teenager, I didn't wish for cars or clothes—I wished that my skin would clear up. I also was extremely frustrated that even though I faithfully used the products and regimens that were marketed to me in my teen magazines and on TV, I never got the results those models got. Of course that's before I knew about having an entourage and the wonders of editing and airbrushing.

I got really good at covering my blemishes with makeup, and I even did my time behind the makeup counters for awhile. It's funny, of all the different jobs and interests I've had in my lifetime, skincare and makeup jobs are where I always seem to return.

I was a stay-at-home mom for years, and it was always my plan to return to work once my kids were in school full-time. There was just one problem...I had no idea what I wanted to be when I grew up! I thought I wanted to be a famous fashion designer in high school. In college, I changed my major three times from Fashion Design to Interior Design to Architecture, and I ultimately graduated with a Bachelor's in Architectural Studies with a minor in Humanities. I knew this degree wouldn't lead me directly to my dream career, but I also didn't want to be in school forever. I had several different jobs in sales, marketing, advertising, and publishing in my twenties, but I never found my one passion—my true purpose. I also knew that whatever career I chose had to have a flexible schedule since I wanted to be present for my children and their activities.

I was discussing this whole scenario with a friend one day while our daughters were having a play date, and she asked me why I didn't just do makeup for weddings and other events, which was always something I had done on the side. I responded that I was concerned about liability issues since I wasn't a licensed cosmetologist or aesthetician, nor was I employed by a makeup company. She looked at me curiously and asked simply, "Well...why don't you just get your license?" And that was it. It was the biggest combination "duh" and "aha!" moment of my life.

I did some research and found a local cosmetology school with a great reputation. I went back to school part time and earned my aesthetics license in 6 months. While I was still in school, I was inspired one day to begin a blog, which would ultimately become my company, my brand, my third child. I began writing it because even though I went back to school so I could be a professional makeup artist, I really fell in love with the skin. I loved the science of skin: biology, histology, physiology, anatomy. I even enjoyed learning about the less intriguing subjects like safety and sanitation, electricity (believe it or not, aestheticians have to learn about different electrical currents), and chemistry—especially cosmetic chemistry and ingredients.

I was fortunate that my teacher believed in a holistic philosophy and taught us topics like the necessity of adequate hydration, proper nutrition, using products that contained safe, natural ingredients and were free of parabens, sulfates, and other potentially harmful chemicals. She also taught us specific triggers to certain skin conditions, for example certain foods that are known to cause acne and broken capillaries, and discussed the importance of probiotics and Vitamin D in maintaining the immune system which ultimately affects skin health. I was so excited about all of this great information that I knew I had to share it. I also started blogging because; you never know... some people get book deals, TV shows, great jobs, or at least free products to try. I knew that finding a job in a spa that fit both my schedule and my holistic skincare philosophy would be tough, so I started writing in an effort to give myself a bit of an edge.

I had one little issue though...I had no idea how to start a blog. I wasn't (and still am not really!) a tech-savvy person. So I bought myself a few of those "...For Dummies" books. Seriously. That's how I learned to blog.

I never did find that perfect spa job with the perfect hours and perfect products and philosophy. What I did do was begin working with clients privately and I continued working on my blog. I also started contributing to trade magazines and other websites. I went through quite a bit of personal transformation during this time as well; I made significant changes in my diet, lifestyle habits, and subsequently (and unexpectedly) lost 80 pounds. Something else amazing happened...my acne went away for good. I was able to ditch the expensive products and start using my own hand-blended natural recipes. I also felt the desire to go back to school again, this time for holistic nutrition. I was already amazed with my own results and had connected the diet and lifestyle changes with the improvement in my skin, so I wanted to learn more. How did this happen? Why did this happen? Was I a unique case or would this work for other people?

As I studied holistic nutrition, I began to realize that most people don't know the information I was learning about how food affects health. It wasn't information commonly taught in many homes, schools, or churches. It's not information that doctors and nurses learn during their education either. Yet, this information not only improved my skin and helped me lose weight, but it also changed my entire life. I had no intention of becoming a holistic health coach. I really intended the holistic nutrition education to be for my own personal knowledge and to establish credibility for writing about nutrition as it pertains to skincare. However, my own experience was so profound and I was so moved by the importance and urgency of the information I was absorbing that I knew I had to use it to help other people experience positive life changes of their own.

I began working with clients while I was still in school under the supervision of my advisor and other staff members. I was amazed that the majority of the people I worked with also began experiencing improvements in their skin conditions during our time together, as well as other wonderful changes like weight loss, blood sugar stabilization, lowered "bad" cholesterol, and improved digestion.

My entire journey —bad skin, lots of jobs, motherhood, going back to school, gaining weight, losing weight, writing my blog, starting my company— is what truly defined that purpose in life that I had hoped would manifest in my early twenties. This was it. Not only was I meant to be a holistic health coach with a focus on holistic skincare, but I was also meant to share my knowledge and experience by continuing to write, teach, and speak in front of large audiences.

You see, going through the process of starting a business, and learning about nutrition literally with actual food and in the more esoteric sense of spiritual nourishment, has been very revealing. When I began coaching my clients, more of my true self was revealed by hearing and feeling their struggles, insecurities, pain, and walking next to them through their triumphs and victories. My journey, and the wonderful gifts that my clients have allowed me to receive by being a part of their journeys, are what really gave me my skin. This new skin is the living, breathing, protector of the vessel (my body), which holds my newly and freely emerging self. Once I learned to look at my whole self in this way, I knew I would never have to hide again—except when I play hide and seek with my kids!

This book will teach you how to have the skin you've always dreamed of without spending a fortune on products or undergoing scary (and risky) procedures like peels, injections, or cosmetic surgery. My knowledge stems from my modern medical aesthetic training, holistic nutrition education and practice (including certifications in health coaching, Ayurveda, and detoxification), experience as an apothecary skincare product formulator and educator, and of course, personal experience. I'll tell you all you need to know about what holistic skincare really is: using nutrition and healthy lifestyle choices in addition to high quality, natural skincare products to nourish and protect the skin from the inside out and outside in. I'll also share more about the process of my own becoming, and how self-acceptance and self-love really paved the way to my own discovery.

If you've ever felt lost, out of touch with yourself, fear that you're not the person you used to be, fear that you're not the person you want to be, then I hope you find some inspiration from my story and know that not only can you have the skin and healthy body that you love (and will love you back), but you can also move forward in your own quest for self-discovery.

# Chapter 1: My Skincare Roller Coaster

Ah, the image of beautiful skin. Supple. Bright. Glowing. Smooth. Radiant. Unmarred. It's the image that comes to mind when watching makeup and anti-aging skincare commercials featuring smiling, dreamy-eyed women who radiate youth and vitality. Of course that image comes crashing down once you buy the product and don't instantly see the same image looking back in the mirror. The idea of beautiful skin has a sound too—like ethereal new age music with raindrops and birds chirping ...and then suddenly, the CD skips or you hit the wrong button on your iPod and a loud death metal song shocks you out of your dreamy state. I know what you're thinking... and the answer is yes the same person can have both new age and death metal on their playlist.

Are these images in the media really achievable by using the advertised products? Or does lighting, professional makeup artistry, editing, and Photoshop really do all the work? I don't know about you, but I certainly don't want to have to have an entourage of makeup artists and lighting crews following me around the grocery store. I'm a real person—a regular wife and working mom. That would just cramp my style! I don't want the crew, but I still want that skin.

To say that growing up with acne was tough is an understatement. I remember being told I had such a pretty face...it was such a shame that it was covered with pimples (or "blemishes" or "zits"—it depends on how politically correct the person was trying to be at the time). Everyone always told me I'd grow out of it: my parents, doctors, friends, even teachers— and I felt extremely cheated that it didn't get better as a young adult. I became the subject of interest of the "mean girls" in school and was teased often. What I didn't realize back then is that the words, sideways glances, snickers, and whispers from those mean girls were no louder and no more damaging than the mean girl in my own mind. It was she who kept me hiding, kept me ashamed, made me use defense as my default response to any situation. It was just easier for me to hear the "real" mean girls so I didn't have to deal with my own issues.

I tried product after product until I finally found a product line that actually worked. I was elated! My skin was completely clear! I ignored the fact that my eyebrows and hairline began to lighten from the constant application of benzoyl peroxide (as did my pillow cases). My skin would hurt (and even sometimes crack) when I smiled and the skin on my face even became several shades lighter than the skin on my neck. I suspected that this was probably not normal, but I was so happy with my newly clear skin, I chose to ignore it.

When I began to follow websites like the Environmental Working Group[1] and the Campaign for Safe Cosmetics[2], I learned about newly published research that definitively linked many of chemicals in the products I used to toxic reactions in the body. I couldn't ignore the dangers of my beloved new products anymore. I was both heartbroken and furious that my savior—the only skincare products that gave me clear skin— contained such harmful chemical ingredients. Heartbroken because I loved my clear skin so much and didn't want to give it up by stopping the products, and furious that those ingredients were even in the products in the first place.

Fortunately, I was in aesthetics school at the time and had access to high-quality products that contained only safe, natural, anti-inflammatory ingredients. I started a regimen with that product line and was able to purchase them with a student discount. This made their cost more comparable with department store brands, but was still a significant increase from the products I stopped using. However, these new products worked! There was a small period of adjustment (which is common for any skin type when switching to a new regimen), but once these new products started working I felt an extreme sense of relief. I would not have to give up my newfound sense of confidence! I also wouldn't have to worry about appearing to be a fraud—after all who wants to go to a pimple-faced aesthetician for skincare treatments and advice? Not me.

My husband and our bank account, however, did not share my enthusiasm since I was now spending the equivalent of a car payment each month on my new products. But I didn't care. I had clear skin and never wanted to go back to the acne-riddled face of my past. I would try something new or less expensive here and there (as an aesthetician and blogger I was never short of free samples), but the acne always returned, mocking me each time. So, I kept paying big bucks for the latest innovations in ingredients and formulations. What I didn't yet realize at the time was that even though I had found products that kept the acne under control on the surface, it never actually went away since I had not addressed the reason it was there in the first place.

# Chapter 2: Weight Affects Skin

I was a skinny kid. I was a skinny teen; I was skinny into young adulthood. After my first child, I lost the baby weight fairly easily and quickly. I even got a big head about it—I confess. I'd see other new moms who couldn't lose their baby weight and am ashamed to admit I had a few mean girl thoughts about them since I was feeling proud of myself for bouncing back into shape so quickly. Little did I know how the tables would turn.

During my second pregnancy I was asked to be a bridesmaid for one of my best friends. The wedding was scheduled six months after my due date and I had a plan. I had been in a wedding for another friend six months after my first pregnancy and I thought I could predict what size I would be based on how soon I'd lost my baby weight the first time. We went bridesmaid dress shopping when I was about seven months pregnant and I was already feeling a little cocky that I could fit into the sample gown pregnant belly and all. I ordered the same size I had ordered for the last wedding, and didn't give it another thought.

Unfortunately for me, things didn't go according to plan. After my second pregnancy, I didn't lose the baby weight at all. I stayed the same weight for awhile, and then I actually began to gain more weight. I couldn't fit into the dress I had ordered, but I refused to admit it.

Though it would've been easy enough to have had the seams let out, this was the age of ephedra—the miraculous weight loss herb. At the time, I thought if it's natural, it must be safe, right? I had read the warnings on the bottle and had heard them in the media but, even though I was a little concerned about the safety, I ignored it just as I ignored my instincts against using those toxic acne products. I was determined to fit into that dress. I also began exercising, mostly doing Pilates. I used this to justify the diet pills because at least exercise was a healthy weight loss effort. I did lose about 15 pounds, but by then, I had sacrificed my mental health. I didn't know then how these pills affect mood and I began to have severe, uncontrollable mood swings. It turns out that none of it was worth the safety risks or mood issues because, despite losing 15 pounds and wearing two pairs of Spanx™, I still didn't fit comfortably into the dress. Oh I got it on, all right. I couldn't breathe or move very well and I was terrified to eat, but I got that thing on. In the wedding pictures, I resembled a stuffed sausage in a burgundy taffeta casing. I felt so guilty that I had ruined the wedding party pictures for the bride, even though she still swears to this day that I looked beautiful.

I continued to gain more weight, and my self-esteem and self-worth plummeted. I no longer cared about makeup and I began wearing oversized, deliberately nondescript clothing. I wanted to hide. There are very few photos of me during that time because I felt so ashamed. The few that do exist show a very sad, scared girl who didn't love herself. The situation became worse as family members began making comments like, "Here, have a salad", or "You don't really need that dessert." Even worse were the family members who would offer me their half-eaten dinners when they were full, assuming that I would finish them.

I became the object of the judgmental mean girl stares everywhere I went. I felt their gazes when I was clothes shopping—even though words were never spoken I heard the thoughts in my head asking if I belonged in this store—shouldn't I be shopping in the plus-size stores? I do believe that negative thoughts and energies can speak louder than words, cutting like a knife, but whether that negativity truly came from other people or whether it was my own self-deprecating, self-loathing thoughts I'm not sure.

Some people hit rock bottom before change can happen—I hit it twice. The first happened when I was window shopping in a department store with my mother. I was wearing my typical unflattering attire and hadn't done my hair or makeup that day. I remember going down the escalator, looking over at the mirrored wall, and the mean girl thoughts entered my head with a vengeance when I saw a girl in the reflection. "Look at that frumpy fat girl. What was she thinking coming to the mall looking like that? I mean yeah, she's fat, but there is no excuse for her to go out like that in public!

She really should put herself together in a way that flatters the figure she has." It took me several seconds to realize that I was that fat, frumpy girl in the reflection.

My second bottom happened around the same time. I can't remember which happened first, but they both had a profound effect on me. I was talking with my sister after a family outing and I began to go into my "woe is me, I'm so fat, nothing I do is working" mode. My sister had heard me say those things before and I guess she had heard enough. My dear sister is a rather direct person. Sometimes she can be overly harsh, but in this case it was pure, tough love. She simply said, "Well, you're clearly not doing enough!"

My jaw dropped. I went on to lament about how I was counting my Points®, logging in my food journal, going to the gym, doing my Pilates, and of course, I had two toddlers who took up the majority of my time. Plus, I had a husband, and did all the shopping, cooking, cleaning…I had every excuse in the book. Her answer: "Well, you aren't doing enough and you aren't doing the right things because if you were, you would have lost the weight by now." That hit me like a ton of bricks. I really hated her for it at the time because it sounded so mean. I didn't speak to her for weeks. Even though it was harsh, maybe even mean, I began to realize that it was the truth—the brutally honest truth.

These two bottoms were my wake-up calls. In one sense, it was very literal. It was the realization that even though I thought I was taking steps to lose the weight, I was either not doing enough or I was doing the wrong thing for my body. Therefore, it was time to start trying something new.

In another sense, this was a spiritual awakening. It was the Universe, God, Divine, Light…whatever you want to call it, slapping me upside the head and yelling "Hello!!!! You are here for a reason! You are meant to do something with your life, and at the very least, you are meant to set a good example for your girls." It was hard, but I took a long, honest look at myself in the mirror and thought, "You know, for whatever reason, you did not lose the baby weight this time like you thought you would. Even though no one else in the family has weight issues, this might just be your body for the rest of your life. You can choose to hate it and hide it, or you can choose to love it and respect it and dress it with pretty clothes, wear makeup again, and do your hair again. The choice is yours."

I made my choice. I would own it. I went through my closet and got rid of all my "skinny" clothes. Saving them had not motivated me to lose weight to fit into them again, and looking at them made me feel emotions of guilt and shame—neither of which would serve me any longer.

I was doing some research about detoxification for a blog post about the skin as a detoxifying organ. I came across a book that looked like it might present detoxification from this particular angle. It turns out I was wrong. I got the book in the mail and opened it to find that it was a diet book. At that point I had tried many diet books and just didn't have it in me to read yet another one. I had come to accept that I was just meant to live out the rest of my life as a curvy, voluptuous woman and I had just gone shopping for new, cute clothes that actually flattered my shape. I didn't want to worry about counting calories or cutting out entire food groups, or depriving myself of foods I loved. If my family wanted me to polish off their leftovers, I was their girl. It was all good.

I decided to read the book anyway—after all, I could always give it away if I didn't like it. Well, this book was not only a keeper, but also my catalyst. It taught me things about digestion, toxic build up in the body, good fats vs. bad fats, that dairy is not, in fact, a food group, the difference between friendly intestinal flora and toxic, pathogenic bacteria and yeasts, food combining, enzymes, the benefits of raw, plant foods, and so much more. I resisted this information at first, because it was still another diet book and I had come so far in my own self-acceptance that I didn't want things to change, even if it was for the better. In hindsight, I realize that my thought process, while somewhat valid, was yet another expression of fear—a highly rationalized defense mechanism.

I remembered that conversation with my sister—that I hadn't been doing enough, or I hadn't done what was right for my body. What this book was suggesting was so far out of my comfort zone that I figured, what the hell? Nothing bad could possibly come from taking probiotics and eating more vegetables and whole grains, right?

It turned out that this book, this particular way of eating, was the key. Now it's certainly not the only book written that teaches these philosophies, but at that time it delivered the message to me in the way I needed to receive it. I lost 10 pounds the very first week. I thought it was a fluke—a figment of my imagination, because my weight had been stabilized at around 200 pounds for several months. I also felt like how I was now eating must be wrong, because it totally contradicted everything I had ever been taught about what was healthy. I also had the constant thoughts in my head that losing weight quickly was not healthy—and it must just be water weight anyway. But the weight continued to come off—it actually seemed to melt off. The chronic digestive issues I had suffered with for years vanished, and I had so much energy I was able to quit my morning and afternoon cups of sugar and whipped cream (with a dash of coffee) cold turkey. My mood drastically improved. If this was the wrong thing for my body, then how was I able to lose weight so quickly and feel this great?

As the weight came off, my skin began to change as well. Even though I was using my luxury skincare products, my skin began to have a new smoothness and radiance. At first, I was a little concerned because I was afraid that the loss of subcutaneous fat (the protective fat layer that lives under the deeper layer of skin) from the weight loss would result in premature aging. My old acne scars did become more visible and my skin appeared thinner, but this did not last long as my body adjusted to the changes. Even though this diet was low in a lot of things, it was rich in high-quality, "good" fats, which helped fortify and moisturize my skin.

I decided to try to wean myself off of the expensive products. I had already begun experimenting with natural ingredients in my kitchen and had come up with several formulas that I thought were really great. I then learned of an opportunity to teach a class at a local neighborhood education organization, and I decided to offer to teach people how to make their own products using my recipes. However, I realized that if I was teaching my students that these basic skincare products were as effective as the ones in the store, I'd better be able to prove it. For the first time in years, I allowed myself to run out of my multiple serums, acne spot treatments, eye creams, lip creams, neck creams, day creams and night creams. I replaced them with my own homemade cleansers, toners, serums, and moisturizers. Though the ingredients were not known to exacerbate acne or clog pores, I was still nervous that I would break out. It didn't happen. In fact, I didn't even have a typical 30-day adjustment period. My skin drank in the nourishing, natural nut butters, plant oils, and essential oils and truly began to glow.

To this day (when this book comes out I will be 36 years old), I still get carded when I order a glass of wine—not all the time—but often enough. Many people do not believe me when I tell them I have an 8-year-old and 6-year-old because they don't think I am old enough to have kids that age.

When asked how I got here—why I do the work that I do, I often explain that I really traveled two different paths, both dependent on the other. I would not have lost the weight if I had not been doing research for a skin article, and my skin would not have permanently improved without the weight loss process that resulted from my change in diet. From this experience, I have learned that "achieving beauty, health, and vitality" really does happen "from the inside out and outside in."

# Chapter 3: The Skin Tells All

I define "holistic skincare" as treating the skin from the inside out and the outside in using nutrition and healthy lifestyle choices in addition to high-quality, natural skincare products to nourish and protect the skin.

Many aestheticians believe that by using non-invasive spa therapies and natural skincare products, they are delivering holistic skincare. Conversely, many holistic and natural health practitioners claim that all one needs to have fabulous, glowing skin is to eat a clean diet, exercise, drink water, meditate, and reduce stress.

It seemed to me that though each side could be right, they also negated each other's merits. Many aestheticians (even holistic ones) are trained to believe that healthy, effective products are all one needs and that while diet and lifestyle are important to support healthy skin, they don't necessarily cause skin to be healthier. On the flip side, many holistic nutrition professionals believe the exact opposite—healthy products are fine for cosmetic reasons but that they are not actually necessary if diet and lifestyle choices are in check. However, after my own skin and diet experience, I began to believe that focusing on BOTH was the way to not only improve the skin, but also improve its health—and by doing so, the results would last much longer.

When we drink water and eat foods that contain nutrients, the internal vital organs are nourished first. By the time it gets to the skin, there's not a lot left. Because the skin essentially gets the leftover nutrients and hydration, it is also important to nourish the skin, protect it, and hydrate it from the outside in with healthy and safe skincare products. That way, you cover all the bases.

While the holistic skincare route might not be as glamorous or dramatic as going to the spa for an expensive new miracle treatment, I believe there are many reasons why it is a better choice. I made it after years of frustration with conventional methods and also after becoming educated on some of the safety concerns with certain product ingredients. However, for me, the best reason to go the holistic route is because your skin is part of your body—it's not some separate entity that requires separate treatment. It is important to consider and treat yourself as a whole person.

Often a skin condition—for example acne, rosacea, psoriasis, eczema, or melasma—is a symptom of something else that might be going on in your health or in other areas of your life. By taking a holistic approach—looking at the diet, lifestyle, and your whole life—rather than just what's visible on the skin's surface, a cause may be found. By identifying and eliminating the cause, you can eliminate the symptom.

It might seem easier and more convenient to take measures to suppress the symptom—whether it's using a steroid for eczema, lasering off visible broken capillaries from rosacea, or taking an antibiotic for acne. However, none of these methods take into account the reason for the condition; and, because that cause is still in the body, the condition could always return …just in time for a special occasion or important presentation at work. Wouldn't it be better if you could just make that fear go away? This is why I believe it should be top priority to do some detective work and find the cause.

**The skin is a window into what's happening inside the body in terms of health.**

We can also examine what's going on emotionally. Are you unhappy, stressed, malnourished, or living with a chronic illness? There is a lot that we can tell just by what's surfacing on the skin, whether it's acne, rosacea, or something more severe like psoriasis. Those are all indications of a condition that might be happening on the inside.

Acne, rosacea, and eczema are all conditions that are connected to the health of the gastrointestinal lining. When I speak with my clients during our initial consultation, we talk a lot about digestion—not just what they are eating, but when they are eating it and how they feel after. Do they experience bloating, pain, reflux, gas, diarrhea, or other symptoms? Usually, it can be assumed that food is not being properly digested. We also talk about how often they go to the bathroom. Not the most fun topics to discuss, but they are relevant.

Here's an amazing statistic: *100% of my clients who have skin conditions also have a digestive issue or food allergy of some kind.* It's really quite staggering. When we address the digestive issues, the skin problems clear up.

Interestingly, Traditional Chinese Medicine (TCM) and Ayurveda (an ancient healing modality from India), both use maps showing how certain areas of the face correspond to certain organs and systems of the body. If you're breaking out on a certain area of your face, you can automatically assume that there is some kind of issue happening in its corresponding organ or system. For example, many women who break out during "that time of the month" get acne around the mouth or chin area. In TCM, this corresponds to the ovaries and the female reproductive system.

What we eat affects every cell of the body, including our skin cells. The quality of the nutrients in the foods we eat are literally the building blocks and raw materials for the new cells that our bodies produce. Those cells form our tissues, organs, and systems—every part of our bodies. The food you eat will determine whether those cells are healthy and vibrant or weak and unhealthy. High-quality, nutrient-dense foods and adequate hydration are the key to nourished, strong skin cells that are not only able to protect and insulate the body, but also give you the beautiful appearance you've always wanted. I always like to say that healthy cells are pretty cells!

**Lifestyle choices are equally as important:**

- Our relationships
- The environmental aggressors or pollutants we live with on a regular basis
- How much exercise we get
- How much stress we have in our bodies

- Our overall outlook on life
- How we take care of ourselves
- How much sleep we get.

Each of these factors has the ability to either facilitate healthy skin production or hinder it.

One question I often hear is, "Who can benefit from holistic skincare?" Many people worry that their skin condition is too severe and can only be helped by conventional means. Some believe too much damage has been done and that harsh treatments, injectable muscle relaxants and dermal fillers, or surgery is their only option. The truth is that holistic skincare can benefit people of any age with any skin condition. There's really nothing bad that can happen by eating better and making healthier lifestyle choices whether you are a teenager undergoing hormonal activity and beginning to break out, or an older woman in menopause experiencing hormonal acne or melasma (a form of hyperpigmentation that happens often in conjunction with increased female hormonal activity). Anyone can benefit from making adjustments to the diet and lifestyle.

According to my colleague, holistic health coach and aesthetician Sharonah Rapseik, PhD: "We must honor the connection between what we see on the outside and what we put into our stomachs, hearts, and minds. Those who can do that experience truly profound improvements in all areas of life."

One of the more controversial questions I often hear is, "Why does my dermatologist tell me that diet has nothing to do with how the skin looks?" That's one of the more frustrating questions for any holistic skincare practitioner. The answer is that it's not really in their training. Doctors and nurses do not get nutrition and lifestyle training in medical or nursing school. They are taught to diagnose based on symptoms and then they are taught how to treat the problem with pharmaceutical drugs or surgery. They are not taught to go deeper into a patient's life and ask what might be going on, or talk about the foods he or she is eating. These healthcare professionals also don't necessarily have the time to spend with their patients to get that full, complete picture of the whole person. It doesn't mean that the dermatologist is necessarily wrong or bad. I certainly don't ever tell people not to go to a doctor. I do inform clients that doctors in general—Western medicine/allopathic doctors—do not receive this information as a part of their education and training, which is why they might say that diet has nothing to do with a particular skin condition.

It's really a difference between a preventative versus reactive approach. A dermatologist reacts to a condition that has already occurred, whereas a holistic practitioner tries to prevent the condition from occurring in the first place. If a condition does occur, a holistic practitioner works to eliminate it for good, rather than simply making it more tolerable with ongoing treatments.

Consider this: doctors see far more sick people than they see healthy people. In fact, most people don't even go to the doctor unless they are already sick. Holistic practitioners in some cultures are not even paid if their patients get sick. Instead, they are paid an annual retainer to keep their patients healthy. If the patients get sick too much that year, the practitioner won't get asked to stick around the next year. It's a very different outlook. Can you imagine if healthcare worked that way?

The good news is that even if someone is already receiving conventional treatment from a doctor, holistic skincare can still be beneficial. While drugs have contraindications and side effects, the majority of fresh, whole foods and most natural skincare ingredients do not!

There's a big misconception that because many natural ingredients are not well known to healthcare professionals, we can't be sure they are safe. For the most part, this is not true. Most essential oils and herbs have been used successfully for thousands and thousands of years with no side effects.

Some do have side effects though, or could react with a conventional synthetic drug—although this is much less frequent than adverse reactions that occur from mixing pharmaceuticals. It's a matter of being educated about what you're using and if you don't know what it is, you must ask a professional knowledgeable in this area, especially if you are already taking a medication and want to add an alternative. Naturopathic or integrative medicine doctors are great resources because they have been trained in conventional medicines as well as herbs, foods, spices, essential oils, and other natural ingredients. They have the most accurate information on what natural remedies can be safely used in addition to pharmaceutical drugs.

In terms of actual products, not medications, it is very important to use common sense. If you do have a reaction to something, you must stop using it and let yourself heal. Read the label to see if you can figure out what the liable ingredient was and try something else—do not use it again. Remember, it is less likely for someone to react to a natural product than it is to react to a chemical product. You're not going to see "dirty dozen" lists with a whole bunch of natural ingredients. Those lists are chock full of ingredients most of us can't pronounce.

While holistic skincare has very few, if any bad side effects, it has lots of good ones! I, as well as many of my clients, have experienced what I like to refer to as "happy side effects." When you clean up your diet, and make changes in your lifestyle, you become healthier on the inside and more balanced overall. You might lose weight, or you might improve your quality of life if you have a chronic illness. I lost 80 pounds and I no longer have to take any pain medication for an old back injury now that I've cleaned up my diet and I follow a strict regimen of yoga, stretching, massages, and inversion. My skin is healthier now than it's been since I was about 10 years old. Nobody believes me when I tell them that I had stage 4 pizza face cystic acne just a few short years ago—nobody.

I personally choose not to take most medications. I believe that there are natural methods that are just as effective, if not more, and certainly have a lot less side effects. However, in the U.S., we have to abide by certain guidelines laid out by the government. I would never tell anyone not to take a prescribed medication. If a client is prescribed a medication that I know to be potentially causative of a side effect, I always encourage the person to research it.

## Vitamin A in Skincare[3]

Isotretinoin, or Accutane®, is a strong oral retinoid used only in the most severe cases of acne. It is a very controversial drug because it is linked to serious side effects and Vitamin A toxicity. It is only prescribed short-term, and Vitamin A blood levels must be regularly monitored during the course of the medication. In my opinion, there are no mild side effects with Accutane. The most common side effects include sudden onset of night blindness, hair loss or alopecia, depression, elevated triglycerides, and liver damage. The list of potential serious side effects is very long, and includes severe birth defects if taken during any part of pregnancy (pregnancy tests are required prior to and during the use of Accutane for female patients), anaphylaxis, psychosis and suicidal tendencies, stroke, seizures, hearing impairment, and more. I have some loyal readers who have taken Accutane with little problems, but I also know of others who have not fared so well.

I do not recommend the use of Accutane for any period of time, or for any reason. I experienced severe pustular and cystic acne (considered to be Grade 4 acne) and am living proof that it can be successfully treated without the use of this drug or any other prescription drugs. Other forms of Vitamin A are much less irritant and still very effective.

I always recommend that people take responsibility for their own health and not just accept what a doctor or any other practitioner, myself included, says is true until they do their homework. We have so many ways to research now that there really is no reason to be putting substances into our bodies without knowing what they are and how they can help. With that said, I certainly make recommendations for diet, nutrition, and lifestyle changes as well as skincare products, which would not interfere with any medication. My strategy would be that by strengthening the person's immune system and getting things balanced in all areas of life, he or she could eventually wean off of that medication, under a doctor's supervision.

Now for the burning question everyone always wants to know: "When will I see results?" The answer is that it depends on several factors and is different for everybody. It depends on the condition and how severe it is. It also depends on the person's existing diet and lifestyle habits—how much actually has to be cleaned up. I think the biggest factor is **how willing a person is to make changes and follow recommendations.** That's huge. I always tell my clients that I can give them all the education and support in the world, but I'm not the one who's going to the grocery store for you. I'm not the one cooking your dinner. I'm not washing your face for you or putting your moisturizer on for you every night. I'm not putting you to bed. Attitude plays a big role.

While skin might not clear up overnight, if a person follows recommendations, it won't take long at all. I saw significant enough results within a month to stay motivated to keep it up. Here's the thing—as you begin to make changes to nutrition and lifestyle, you will start to see results. You will start to feel great and look great. You're not going to want to go back to habits or substances that set you back before. Once you find what works for you in a diet and balance in your life, you won't want to go back.

You also have to be willing to be adaptable—our bodies change as we age. I know this seems obvious, but I see so many women who have had the same skincare regimen for 20 years and wonder why it's no longer working. You have to be willing to make adjustments as your environment and body change over time. If you do this, you can see positive results with your skin for the rest of your life

Holistic skincare can treat many skin conditions such as acne, rosacea, eczema/dermatitis, and psoriasis. These conditions usually stem from similar causes, which is why it is usually easier to manage them holistically. Other skin conditions that can be successfully managed holistically are keratosis pilaris, fungal rashes (often caused by yeast overgrowth), melasma, and other types of hyperpigmentation (dark spots that appear on the face). Certain signs of premature aging—fine lines and wrinkles—can also be improved. Holistic skincare nourishes and fortifies the skin from the inside out so it can hold itself up better and is less likely to sag. Also, skin tends to thin as it ages. Eating enough of the right nutrients will help to plump up the skin and slow down the progression of aging.

**It is important to keep expectations realistic.**

Holistic skincare isn't going to turn back the hands of time or "erase" wrinkles or scars. Certain damage, like severe burns, deep scars, or extreme sun damage cannot be undone with holistic skincare alone. For example, if a 90-year-old woman who was out in the sun her whole life never using sunscreen comes to me with sun spots and intense, static wrinkles, there's not a lot I can do for her with just diet, lifestyle, and products. She might experience some improvement in the appearance of her skin. By building up the skin underneath, we might be able to plump some of that out; but typically, when that much damage has been done, the only intervention that would make a significant improvement would be a medical intervention, which, of course, would come with risks.

In general, though, when you really take care of yourself from the inside out and pamper and nourish the skin from the outside in, you're going to enjoy beautiful and long-lasting results.

Some results that my clients have experienced since treating their skin from the inside out and outside in include:

- Significant improvement or complete resolution of acne
- Significant reduction in flare-ups of rosacea, eczema, psoriasis, and keratosis pilaris (AKA "chicken skin" on backs of arms, thighs, buttocks)
- Reduced undereye circles and puffiness
- Improvement in pigmentation/evenness of tone
- Overall brighter, more youthful skin—diminished lines and wrinkles
- Improvement in overall texture and the appearance of scars

### The hormone connection

Acne is often caused by hormones. When boys and girls start to get acne during puberty and all kinds of crazy things are going on in their minds and bodies, their skin starts to change as oil glands start to produce more oil. Sweat glands begin to get more active, and start to detoxify more through the skin.

It's a fairly well-known fact that teens aren't the healthiest eaters either. When they go out with their friends, they are not going out to five-star restaurants. When you add the chemicals, sugar, salt, and grease from these food-like substances (sorry, but teenage junk food is not food!) to high hormonal activity, skin conditions are much more likely to erupt.

During pregnancy and menopause women often experience skin changes as well. Melasma is quite common during pregnancy (which is why it was given the nickname "pregnancy mask"), menopause, and when taking certain hormones like birth control pills. During these times of life, women who have had perfect skin their entire lives might begin to experience sudden and severe skin changes and may become completely frustrated by that. Fortunately, many foods and natural remedies have the ability to balance out the hormone levels and are safe to take during pregnancy.

### Why did this happen to me?

Many times, a person with a skin condition asks the challenging question, "Why was I affected with this but my sister has perfect skin?" There is no single answer to that question. Some people blame genetics, but it's actually my belief (which is supported by others) that while genetics can be somewhat of a blueprint for a health or skin condition, it's not necessarily a sentence.

So, if your mom had really bad acne and ate poorly, and you also eat poorly, you are likely to suffer from acne too. But if you eat really healthy and make different lifestyle choices, there is a strong possibility that you might not get acne because you're changing one of the variables in the equation. How people eat and what lifestyle choices they make have more of an impact than genetics alone.

## Holistic skincare is a lifestyle change

In order to truly get lasting results inside and out, we need to let go of the "Band-Aid®" mentality. Our Western medicine society has trained us to pop pills for almost anything to make symptoms go away. Rarely do we think to find the reason why we are uncomfortable. We just cover it up—put the blinders on. Holistic skincare is very different from this obsession with quick fixes, miracle pills, fad diets, get-rich-quick schemes, and become skinny overnight juices. "Quick" is just not the way true healing happens.

The body is more than capable of healing itself if it is given everything it needs One of those requirements is time. It takes the body a little while to adjust to a new diet and skincare regimen and also to let go of some of the toxins and damage it's been holding on to. If you give your body what it needs in terms of nutrients and a healthy lifestyle, it will thank you for it. Your skin will thank you for it. Your skin will reflect it. It just might take time depending on how much damage has been done.

If you want good results, you're going to have stick with it, otherwise you may wind up adding back certain foods, substances, or lifestyle choices that contributed to the problem in the first place and it will come back again. So you have to make the decision. Do you want to have nice skin and look great? Or do you want to have breakouts and possibly gain weight or get sick just so that you can enjoy certain vices that might not be serving you? It's a personal decision, but if you commit to it and stick with it, it will benefit you for your whole life.

## Are you ready to get started?

There are so many aspects to holistic skincare that a person who is ready and willing really can jump in anywhere. A great way to start is to begin adding more fresh fruits and vegetables into the diet. Another simple thing to do is to start drinking more water. It's also a really good idea to read the labels on the skincare products you already have and see how many of the ingredients you can pronounce. Look them up on the Environmental Working Group's Skin Deep® Cosmetics Database[4] to see how they score in terms of safety (heads up—what you see might alarm you). There are quite a lot of other resources available on the Internet. I always recommend that people read up on nutrition, TCM, and Ayurveda. These methods have a lot of information about how the skin correlates with internal health, diet, and nutrition.

Any small change in the right direction is progress. You may also consider working with someone like me who has been trained in this field. That person has already read the books and done the research. He or she already tried the different products, and knows what works. A holistic practitioner can help guide people based on where they are in their lives and on their journeys.

# Chapter 4: Will People Think I'm Vain?

So many people believe that having a regular skincare regimen and/or wearing makeup is vain. I had a hard time with this myself because I began wearing a lot of makeup at a very young age to cover my acne. There seems to be an insidious misconception that wanting to be beautiful means you are a shallow or superficial person. This couldn't be further from the truth!

No one wonders why someone looking at a beautiful, perfect flower would marvel at its perfection. What about admiring a beautiful work of art in a museum or being captivated by the music of the symphony? You don't ever hear people say, "Wow, she is so vain for appreciating all of that beauty." Why can't we want and enjoy the beauty of our own physical bodies? We are one of the first people we see every day when we look in the mirror. Why shouldn't we want the first images we see to be beautiful? Why shouldn't we want one of the last images we see before going to bed to be beautiful as well?

There is nothing wrong with wanting to look and feel beautiful. Human beings are naturally drawn to that which is beautiful—if that wasn't true, no one would have dedicated their lives to creating epic, timeless works of art, music, drama, or architecture. We wouldn't decorate our homes, offices, or yards with ornaments and pictures or paintings. Why is it so horrible to want to decorate yourself? Many cultures around the world have long histories of adornment rituals commemorating special moments or rites of passage in a woman's life. Their histories are much older than our nation's Puritanical values.

We are taught that seeking beauty equates to seeking excess. So many of us care about how we are perceived by others. Unfortunately, we have to—whether we want to admit it or not, people do judge based on our appearance. It almost seems like you can't win, right? If you go out of your way to present yourself well and make a good impression, someone might call you vain. I've been there.

There was a point in my own journey where I kind of gave up on myself because I really thought that nothing was working—I just gave up. I went from people thinking that I was vain because I wore a lot of makeup and obsessed about my skincare routine to people thinking that I was a slob because I stopped.

I eventually realized that people will judge you no matter what because everybody has their own issues going on. I learned that it's never about me, it's always about them. People view the world and other people through their own perspective, which is influenced by their own experience.

So if people think that you are vain because you are taking better care of yourself and focusing more on your skin I say fuhgeddaboutit! Let others think whatever they want because it's just their way of expressing or covering up an insecurity about their own. No matter what actions we take, we will never have control over how others perceive us. We only have control over ourselves.

Taking care of yourself and believing you look good lifts your spirits. People get busy, or sick, give birth, or endure a negative experience such as a death in the family or getting fired. Often, they allow these events to give them an excuse to let themselves go. New moms especially are very prone to this, and reasonably so. After giving birth, a woman is exhausted and overwhelmed. She's so busy taking care of the baby and adjusting to her new life and identity that she lets herself go. After I gave birth to my kids, I didn't even want to look in the mirror because my body was so different and my face had changed—even my nose looked different. I didn't even recognize myself and instead of fixing myself up a bit (after the initial haze passed—let's be realistic here!) I allowed myself to get into a negative mindset that gave me permission to hide. I was sad at a time when I should have been full of joy.

Another scenario is the aging woman who misses how she once looked, or a woman going through a hard time who remembers much happier days. People associate how they looked at various times in their life with certain lifestyles they once had or when times were easier.

When you're feeling down, it really does a body good to just freshen up a bit. Take a hot shower, wash your face, brush your hair, maybe add a little makeup—I'm not saying you have to put a full face on—especially if you are a new mom and not quite awake. Just put in a little effort and I promise you will feel better than if you had thrown your hair in a sloppy ponytail, pulled on your ratty sweatpants, and left the house with crusts in your eyes!

Sometimes, it's hard to snap out of frumpy mode. I've been lucky to have people in my life to gently—well, not always gently—nudge me back in the right direction. I have a friend who I worked with when I was in my early 20s. My nails were always done, I always had makeup on, and my hair was perfect and shiny. Years later, we ran into each other. I had no makeup on, my hair looked crazy, my oldest daughter was 2-years-old—I was in full mommy mode. She gaped at me when she saw me. "Rachael is that you?" With nowhere to run, I finally admitted it was me. I was so ashamed of my appearance. After some small talk, she said "Rachael it's so weird seeing you without your hair and makeup done! That's just not like you!" That really hit home for me. No, it wasn't me. I did enjoy wearing makeup and fixing myself up. Caring about your appearance means you care about yourself. Appreciating your own inherent beauty means you appreciate your own special talents and unique gifts.

I think that most women are very devoted to caring for other people: spouses, children, co-workers, friends, parents, siblings. Whether we're mothers or not, we're nurturers and givers. It's engrained in many of us to give to others first and put ourselves last. This is a lifestyle change that I really enjoy working on with people. Shifting some focus back onto you, letting yourself enjoy a spa treatment or day of pampering without any guilt. Think of it as a well-deserved reward for being a giving, generous, nurturing woman.

## How can spa treatments help the skin?

It depends on the condition, but several spa treatments are not just for pampering, beautification, and relaxation; they can be very therapeutic. Spa treatments can help soothe and calm irritated skin, tone facial muscles, and boost the skin's ability to detoxify. These include full-body treatments such as salt or sugar scrubs, dry brushing, body wraps, and hydrotherapy. Salt baths and mud baths are very helpful for drawing out toxins through the skin. Some of the scrubs and massages encourage lymphatic drainage, which also helps detoxification. While many treatments are beneficial, remember there's nothing wrong with pampering either!

People with acne, rosacea, or another inflammatory condition must use caution when considering spa treatments. It is very important to do your research on the type of spa you want to visit because many aestheticians were trained to treat these conditions too aggressively with exfoliation. I do not believe in causing additional friction or inflammation to an already inflamed skin condition.

Soothing masks, mists, and creams contain cooling, calming ingredients that help heal inflammatory conditions. For acne, there are also certain cleansing and facial massage procedures that can help expel dirt out of the pores without stripping out oils or damaging surrounding tissue. It is important to talk to your aesthetician and ask about her exfoliation philosophy.

# Self Care is Not Selfish[5]

Many people, moms and those who care for others on a regular basis, often prioritize the needs of others above their own. I get it. I have kids, and I have clients. I care deeply about my friends and family. Their level of happiness affects my own. It's just the way I am.

It's important to remember though, that you can't effectively take care of others if your own needs are not being met. Even though I work in aesthetics and wellness, I still need to remind myself to make sure my own needs are taken care of. I can't function as effectively or efficiently if I don't.

### What is self-care?

I believe that self-care is an upgraded version of daily living. It is a way to add pleasure to an otherwise mundane day, and to make yourself feel good just because. I want to be clear that self-care does not equate to narcissism and does not mean ignoring responsibilities to others—there has to be a balance. But as days get busy and tasks, appointments, and other obligations begin to pile up, we often sacrifice important things like sleep, good food, love, affection, hygiene, and relaxation. But omitting these from our lives raises stress hormone levels and forces the body into survival mode. This leads to many chronic problems like digestive issues, skin problems, and inflammation. I encourage you to make a conscious decision every day to take care of yourself in at least one way.

### 8 simple ways to improve your self-care.

1.  **Daily affirmations.** When you wake up every morning, take a nice, long stretch and say to yourself, "Today is a wonderful day."

2.  **Wear clothes that make you feel attractive and confident every day,** even if you are just running out for errands. This is not to please other people. This is so that when you catch a glimpse of

yourself in windows or mirrors, YOU feel good.

3. **Breathe.** Deep, deliberate breathing has been scientifically proven to reduce the effects of stress on the body.

4. **Go to a spa.** If you have stiff joints or sore muscles, book a massage. If you feel you are looking puffy or your skin is breaking out, get a facial. If money is tight, you can still enjoy a spa experience with a relaxing and inexpensive manicure or pedicure.

5. **Drink tea.** Drink high-quality teas with locally made, raw honey. White and green teas are very low in caffeine, are rich in antioxidants, and help the body detoxify. Other varieties like rooibos and herbal teas contain no caffeine or other stimulants. They relax the mind and soothe the senses with their wonderful aromas. I prefer my tea warm—it is easier on the digestive system than iced.

6. **Cook most of your meals from scratch.** Cooking healthy, good food does not have to be complicated or expensive. Choose simple, fresh ingredients and use seasonings that you like. A well-prepared, simple homecooked meal trumps a restaurant meal nutritionally any day.

7. **Leave early.** Did you ever have one of those days where you are rushing to get somewhere and it seems like you hit every single red light, get stuck in traffic, or crawl behind slow-moving vehicles? I noticed that I never have those days when I am running early. So don't try to squeeze in that last phone call, email, or blog post (note to self)—it can wait until you return. You will feel much better if you have time to spare by being early rather than trying to simply be on time.

8. **Sleep!** This is my biggest challenge, and it is my biggest priority for my own self-care. I tend to work late, and afterward, I feel

the need to read, watch, or play on Facebook to unwind before bed. I rarely get to bed before midnight. This is bad! The body needs sleep to rest and regenerate. Sleep is also the only time the body is not producing cortisol—a stress hormone. It's the only chance the body and mind have to NOT endure physical and emotional stress. Sleep is not a luxury, it is a necessity.

**A word of caution: Not all spa treatments are safe.**

I do not believe in aggressive exfoliation techniques like chemical peels or microdermabrasion. A lot of spas are really pushing these treatments now because they can charge a lot for them and the demand is high. This is where my philosophy differs from many conventional aestheticians, and is the main reason why I choose not to work in a spa. It's hard to find one that shares my non-invasive, inside out-outside in philosophy and uses products that I'd be comfortable standing behind.

These treatments are often indicated for resurfacing, anti-aging, and even to treat acne, rosacea, eczema, and keratosis pilaris. When I used to do those procedures on my own clients, I found it caused more damage than good. Clients who had been getting these treatments for a long time had thinner, more fragile, less elastic skin than clients with similar profiles who did not receive those treatments.

I also noticed more broken capillaries on those clients, especially those who got a lot of microdermabrasion, because that treatment involves suction as well as abrasion of the skin. This is a very damaging combination because it's causing inflammation and it's also pulling up the blood vessels from underneath the skin. Breaking blood vessels in the skin like this can be permanent.

When I was in aesthetics school, we worked on each other to complete all of our required hours for each procedure in the allotted time. At one point,

I was getting microdermabrasion and chemical peels every week, and I graduated with broken capillaries and lines on my forehead that weren't there when I started. In my opinion, those treatments may make the skin look firmer and plumper at first, but once the effects wear off, you are left with more damage that may be irreparable.

**If these treatments are not safe, why do so many women pay an arm and a leg for them?**

Chemical peels, also referred to "chemical exfoliation" come in varying degrees of strength. The superficial, or "lunchtime peel" is a big trend, because a woman can go to the spa on her lunch hour and get a treatment without appearing to have any damage or needing the healing time required after a deeper or medical-strength peel. Deeper peels cause extreme redness, swelling, oozing, and peeling. They're also quite painful and often require anesthesia.

After a lunchtime peel, a woman might be just a little pink and sensitive. Her skin will be plumper and more youthful looking. Lines are often minimized, and she will have a glow. What she doesn't realize is that it's not actually a "healthy glow" with fresh new skin cells brought to the surface, which is how peels are advertised. The glow is actually swelling– edema –injury and inflammation. Peels are popular because you do look really nice after the procedure. But to keep that look, you must do them often. Most protocols suggest one treatment per week for 6 weeks, and then once a month for maintenance. That racks up a lot of money and causes so much inflammation to the skin that it often cannot repair fast enough.

Even if you're not getting microdermabrasion or chemical peels, you've most likely tried a scrub, or spinning cleansing brush. We're often told that these products slough off dead skin cells, revealing healthy, youthful cells underneath. I believe that the skin keeps the dead cells (called corneocytes) as part of its armor as long as they're needed before it sloughs them off naturally. When you force the skin to slough itself sooner than it's ready to, you make the skin more susceptible to injury, infection, inflammation, and damage from the sun and elements. I'm not opposed to a very light enzyme cleanser or mask at home—I'm just not a fan of using exfoliation like sandpaper and treating the face like a splintery board.

# Chapter 5: Healthy Skin is Beautiful Skin

It's important to understand the whole purpose of the skin and its role in health. There is a huge misconception that skincare is all about using expensive products to appear younger or that going to the spa is frivolous and only for the pampered. In reality, the appearance and care of the skin has a direct relationship to overall health and wellness.

Improving one's health can improve the skin, but believe it or not this is true conversely as well. The skin is an important part of the body's immune system. One of its most important functions is to protect the body, particularly the internal organs. The skin is like our coat of armor that shields us from the sun's harmful UV rays, and also keeps unhealthy bacteria and microbes, environmental pollutants, and other invaders out. Protection is only one of the skin's many jobs, and if it's not cared for properly, it won't be a strong barrier.

The skin is held together by a matrix of different proteins, cells, sebum (the oil produced by the sebaceous glands) sweat (produced by the sudoriferous glands), and various other cells, fluids, and lipids. This matrix is called the acid mantle. If we're dehydrated, use harsh products, experience prolonged exposure to the sun or other elements, break out in acne, a rash, eczema, or have other eruptions and areas of compromised and broken skin, it's easier for bacteria and viruses to enter the body. The more intact the skin's barrier, the better it can keep invaders out and our inner systems healthy.

Practicing good skincare habits is one of the best ways to keep the skin's barrier function intact and functioning properly. Symptoms such as dryness, flaking, redness, or itching often indicate the skin's barrier function is damaged. This by far is the most important reason to take care of your skin.

The skin also plays a big role in our sense of touch. It's a sensory organ containing nerve endings. Our skin is how we come into contact with different people and in addition, the skin helps to regulate body temperature.

**Of course, there are aesthetic reasons to take care of the skin as well.**

In an informal survey I conducted as part of my preparation for this book, out of 96 respondents, *more than 62% said their skin appeared brighter and more youthful after following a good skincare product regimen and making healthful changes in diet and lifestyle.* When the skin's condition is at its best, you don't have to apply as much make up, and the makeup you do wear goes on more evenly, looks better, and lasts longer.

**Here are two ways you can improve the appearance of your skin without leaving your house:**

1. **Facial massage.** Massage helps tone and firm up the skin and keeps it from sagging. There are many quick techniques you can try to give yourself a facial massage at home. I incorporate a quick chin and neck massage right into my product application technique. It takes no extra time and it has made a really big difference in my own chin and neck appearance (double chins run in my family—no joke). You can learn this simple technique by watching this video on my YouTube channel[6]: http://www.youtube.com/watch?v=FgCznEXagNQ

2. **Sleep on your back.** Many people don't like to sleep on their backs but when you are sleeping on one side, the compression of the skin into the pillowcase can cause fine lines and wrinkles over time. When you sleep on your side, gravity's working against you. Sleeping on your back, however, can make a big difference. Think of it as gravity giving you a facelift over time!

**I don't like the terms "anti-aging" or "age management".**

We're all aging—there's nothing we can do about it. We can try to "manage" it, but even then, nature doesn't always comply. We might as well just go with it, right? That doesn't mean that aging has to be a bad thing. It can be a beautiful thing and it is nothing to be ashamed of.

The skin does lose moisture as we age, so proper hydration is very important on the inside and on the outside. I often tell clients to keep a little bit of toner or rose water in their purses and spritz it on the face throughout the day. It's wonderful if you're feeling a little bit tired, dehydrated, or even just to freshen up a little. Hydration is very important to preventing the early signs of aging as well as protecting the skin from the sun and the elements. Once the skin is hydrated, it is also important to seal that moisture in with a nourishing and protecting moisturizer. This will fortify the skin's acid mantle and prevent trans-epidermal water loss (TEWL).

"Anti-aging" spa treatments are all the rage these days, and come in a variety of different types from holistic to invasive medical therapies. I prefer noninvasive treatments that have proven results in before-and-after pictures such as LED and microcurrent. Don't worry, it's not as scary as it sounds. Microcurrent releases a very small amount of alternating current in a concentrated area and actually retrains the facial muscles to firm up instead of sag. Ultrasound therapy is another noninvasive, yet effective treatment that offers similar benefits. The LED light stimulates collagen and elastin production in the deeper layers of the skin and doesn't have any side effects. I actually use a handheld LED light at home.

Another holistic—though somewhat invasive— treatment is facial or cosmetic acupuncture. Cosmetic acupuncture uses traditional acupuncture methods to specifically target specific points on the face. In TCM, as well as in Ayurveda, different areas of the face correspond to different organs[7] and systems of the body. According to these philosophies, lines, puffiness, or wrinkles that appear on the face are clues to what is going on internally. Specifically, these facial problems may signify blockages, toxic build-up, or may indicate an organ or system is not functioning optimally. The theory is that inserting needles into these various points and on the face will help unblock/re-balance the corresponding organs or systems, and in doing so will resolve the lines/wrinkles on the face.

Other theories suggest that the needles trigger the cells in the dermis (the deepest layer of the skin where most skin aging occurs) to produce more collagen and elastin (the proteins of youth), giving the skin a plumper, smoother, more youthful look. This theory has been incorporated into one of the newer, and somewhat controversial medical aesthetic techniques called microneedling which I don't recommend.

**Textural concerns are very common.**

They often include scars, uneven moisture in the skin (areas of extreme dryness and oiliness), or large pores. People with naturally oilier skin tend to have large pores, and many wish they didn't because they tend to attract and retain visible debris that can later develop into acne. I encourage these women to embrace their large pores and oily skin! Oilier, thicker, larger-pored skin actually shows signs of aging slower and is more resilient to the effects of the sun as well as environmental aggressors. It might be more prone to acne, but proper skincare will control this condition.

There is some confusion about "minimizing" pore size. Many products claim they can "shrink pores or reduce pore size," but in actuality, this is impossible. Pores aren't muscles. They don't expand and contract. They're openings that allow for hair growth and secretion of sebum and sweat. Following a good cleansing regimen is a good way to minimize the appearance of large pores because if debris and dead skin cells accumulate and become impacted, they'll expand even more. As the debris inside becomes oxidized, the pores will begin to darken, making them more prominent. If you wear makeup, you can try a primer after you cleanse, which will create a barrier over the opening of the pores, making them less noticeable.

**Makeup for skin conditions**

I'm often asked how much makeup should be worn if a person has a skin condition. Doesn't makeup clog pores? Won't using brushes and applicators spread bacteria and make acne worse? Won't the ingredients in the makeup cause allergic or irritant reactions for people with rosacea or eczema? This is a personal choice, and yes, choosing, applying, and storing the products and applicators must all be done carefully.

Because of my acne, I started wearing makeup at a very young age—and not just lip gloss and eyeshadow. I wore full-face concealer and foundation. At one point, I even tried green pigment under my foundation because I thought it would counteract the red of the acne. It did work, but it was quite a hassle and time consuming to blend the foundation in with the green so I didn't end up looking like the Wicked Witch of the West.

I later discovered that those products were also filled with heavy synthetic oils and dyes that block and suffocate the skin, preventing it from breathing and healing. Most of the ingredients clogged pores and contained irritants, which made my acne worse.

Fortunately, there are several high-quality, professional makeup lines available from salons, spas, and online that don't contain these heavy, irritating, and asphyxiating ingredients. For those with erupted, irritated skin, I typically recommend products with healing ingredients, natural pigments, and without comedogenic (pore-clogging) ingredients such as isopropyl myristate, isostearic acid, and coal tar (often a component of dyes). It's important to note that natural emollients such as lanolin, coconut oil, olive oil, and cocoa butter are also comedogenic, though they are soothing for skin types that don't experience breakouts.

In terms of makeup application, I like to use a concealer to spot-treat any blemishes, followed by a tinted moisturizer or mineral powder foundation on top. Mineral powders cover well and you don't need a lot. They are quick and easy to apply, and they allow the skin to breathe without clogging pores. I don't recommend heavy liquids or creams for people with inflammatory skin conditions, although some aestheticians and camouflage makeup artists do use them.

Using makeup to cover rosacea is a little different from covering acne because it's more widespread and it may or may not be accompanied by acne. There is a form of acne, called "acne rosacea" that can accompany rosacea, but sometimes, rosacea appears only as redness, irritation, and broken capillaries. If there's no acne present, but you want to neutralize redness and cover capillaries, you might need a little more makeup or even a little bit of camouflage makeup, which is a highly pigmented and more opaque form of concealer or foundation. Camouflage makeup is useful for scarring and other textural issues which might be present as well. Again, I recommend purchasing these products from a professional source. The makeup sold at drug stores and even department stores contain low-quality ingredients that are often toxic. Most of the time, these won't make the condition better, and might actually make it worse. Remember–it's not about how much makeup to apply, it's more about what kind of makeup to use.

It's a great idea to learn proper application techniques from an aesthetician or makeup artist knowledgeable about ingredients and camouflaging skin conditions, rather than simply going to a department store makeup counter.

# Chapter 6: Detoxification and Skincare

The characteristic that I enjoy talking about the most regarding the skin is detoxification and elimination—I know, weird, right? Most people don't share my enthusiasm for detoxification and elimination, but these are very important topics—vital to overall health, actually. The skin eliminates toxins from the body via the sweat glands. It's very important not to inhibit sweating. When we sweat, we're ridding our bodies of junk, just like we do when we go to the bathroom. We wouldn't apply a product to inhibit urination or defecation just for convenience, would we? However, we have no problem applying anti-perspirants (most of which contain aluminum and other harmful substances) and regulate room temperatures so that we don't sweat because we don't want to smell or stain our clothing. However, when we inhibit sweating, toxins are pushed back into the body where they can accumulate and make us sick. So let them out! If you don't want to sweat on a regular basis because you have to be around people, then turn on your air conditioner, but then it's a good idea to regularly sit in a sauna or hot shower to let your skin detoxify in a controlled environment.

The more the skin can do to eliminate toxins, the less the other organs have to do. Every organ in the body has multiple functions. The organs in the body most responsible for detoxification are the skin, kidneys, colon, and liver. These organs are often overloaded, especially the liver because it filters everything that comes into the body. Most of us are under so much stress physically and we come into contact with so many toxins from the environment, poor diet (resulting in underdigested foods), and toxins that our own bodies produce that many people suffer from liver malfunction which may lead to failure.

### About detoxification

Detoxification is a buzzword we hear a lot these days. Detoxification, sometimes referred to as "internal cleansing" is the process of removing built up toxins from the body. It can be achieved through cleansing diets, cleansing supplements, salt baths body wraps, colonics, and even fancy machines that pull the toxins out of your body through your feet. These different techniques are designed to assist the body's natural process of removing toxic buildup through the liver, kidneys, lungs, lymphatic system, and skin.

Detoxification helps all of the organs and body systems function properly so that the body can properly eliminate toxins. Due to stress, poor diet, lack of exercise, and poor lifestyle choices like smoking and excessive alcohol use, the body accumulates more toxins than it can eliminate on its own. These toxins build up in the body and cause many serious problems such as illness, disruption of essential body functions like digestion, and skin problems such as:

- Acne
- Eczema or dermatitis
- Allergic reactions like rashes or hives
- Signs of premature aging like fine lines and wrinkles
- Seborrhea
- Rosacea
- Psoriasis
- Keratosis pilaris
- Melasma and other forms of hyperpigmentation.

My first experience with detoxification occurred on a cruise ship spa when I was on my honeymoon. This wasn't my first trip to the ship's spa—it was probably my third or fourth! I was having such a wonderful time pampering myself with facials, scalp massages using exotic oils, reflexology pedicures, you name it.

I know what you're thinking—why was I spending so much time in the spa on my honeymoon? Wasn't I supposed to be spending time with my husband? Don't worry, we had an awesome time together. We ate wonderful meals, went on a helicopter tour over the Virgin Islands, boarded a submarine and went down 100 feet to the ocean floor. We visited a butterfly farm, shopped 'til we dropped, and just enjoyed ourselves. However, like on most cruises, there were many activities and excursions available to suit just about every interest. So while my husband was off enjoying one of these, I would go to the spa.

By day 3 or 4, I had already tried most of the basic treatments and was ready to get a little more adventurous with the spa menu. One of the staff members tried to entice me with an escape pod-type device that allegedly relaxed the body so much that it was equivalent to a full night's sleep. While it was intriguing, I passed. Instead, I chose a treatment called Ionithermie®, which was meant to help me lose inches and get rid of cellulite by covering my body with blue clay and then zapping me with electrodes for 30 minutes to break up the toxins in my fat cells. Doesn't that sound like something you'd like to try on your honeymoon? Looking back, I can't help but wonder what the heck was I thinking?

Anyway, I lost inches and my skin did look smoother. During the treatment, I picked the aesthetician's brain and learned all about the different layers of the skin and how toxins get stored in the fat cells. She explained how subcutaneous fat cells (called adipose tissue) expand when full of toxins and become hard and plump like grapes. The electrical current broke up those "grapes" so the toxins could be circulated through the lymphatic system and then eliminated. She convinced me to buy some herb and mineral supplements and told me to drink large amounts of water to help flush out the toxins.

I followed this treatment with a series of mineral-soaked compression body wraps when I got home. These wraps use compression to "squeeze" the toxins from the adipose tissue—kind of like juicing grapes to make wine. In this case, my toxins came out of my hands and feet, and were caught in plastic bags. It was absolutely disgusting—the feeling of the wet bandages, the color and smell of the toxins—but I also found it fascinating.

I didn't continue these expensive treatments because of course, the "inches" came back even though I drank water and took supplements as instructed. However, the fascination stuck with me through the years as I began to learn more about the skin as a detoxifying organ in aesthetics school and while studying yoga and Ayurveda.

## What are toxins?

Toxins are chemicals or substances that are created as a byproduct of the body's processes or when foods don't get digested properly. Toxins also result from exposure to external elements and substances that enter the body through the skin via inhalation or while eating or drinking. These substances include pesticides, synthetic fragrances, artificial additives like preservatives and dyes, chlorine from drinking, swimming, or showering in chlorinated water, and so on. These substances provide no benefit to the body, and the body does not recognize them or know what to do with them. Therefore, they accumulate and can become dangerous, negatively affecting every system of the body.

If you imagine a functioning machine with a bunch of pipes, the toxins are the gunk that gets stuck in there and causes blockages. They can accumulate and harden, become encrusted in the colon, and begin to ferment and rot, preventing the body from eliminating properly. The toxins become putrid and begin to breed parasites, feed harmful strains of bacteria and yeast, and cause internal inflammation. They also get stored in the fat cells, which lie directly underneath the skin, and contribute to cellulite.

If toxins cannot be properly released through the different elimination channels, they get forced further up the intestinal tract, deeper into the body. The toxins can cause diseases and conditions, including skin conditions. Biochemist and president of Beyond Health International, Raymond Francis writes in his book, Never Be Sick Again[8], that there are really only two causes of disease: deficiency and toxicity. The toxins prevent the body from producing healthy cells that perform healthy functions.

This fact is the main reason to detoxify. We want the body to function properly and to produce healthy cells. The more we can do facilitate the body's natural process of detoxification, the better off we will be.

The skin is a detoxifying organ. When we eat healthier foods, use healthier products on the skin and in the home, and limit exposure to harmful substances and environmental pollutants, we lower the chance that toxins will show up on the skin as a condition like acne or rosacea.

**What foods naturally help the body detoxify?**

- Organic plant foods that are naturally high in enzymes and fiber are the most detoxifying foods. Some examples are:
- Dark green lettuces and dark leafy greens like spinach, romaine, and dandelion greens
- Crucerifous greens like broccoli, kale, and Brussels sprouts
- Sea vegetables like nori, kombu, and wakame
- White and green tea are also very detoxifying
- Whole grains like quinoa and brown rice
- Fresh, raw fruits and vegetables
- Beans and legumes
- Raw, soaked nuts and seeds
- Fermented foods like kefir, raw sauerkraut, kim chi, and other cultured vegetables.

**Why are organic or locally sourced foods preferred?**

Organic foods are healthier because they have fewer toxins. Most people are aware that conventionally farmed produce contains residues of herbicides, insecticides, and pesticides. They also contain other synthetic chemicals that are used to increase the crop yields and size of the crops, as well as to force them to ripen after they are prematurely harvested. In addition, conventional produce is much more likely to be grown from genetically modified seeds. A genetically modified or engineered food is "a plant or meat product that has had its DNA artificially altered in a laboratory by genes from other plants, animals, viruses, or bacteria, in order to produce foreign compounds in that food. This type of genetic alteration is not found in nature, and is **experimental**.[9]"

It's even worse with conventionally raised animal products. Cruelty issues aside, many people—myself included—have significantly reduced their intake of animal products because of the hormones, antibiotics, and other synthetic chemicals that these foods contain. The animals live in overcrowded and highly unsanitary conditions where infections and injuries are common. Therefore, the animals are regularly treated with antibiotics. Furthermore, they are fed unnatural diets because it is cost effective and fattens them up faster. Finally, these animals are administered growth hormones to increase size, as well as milk and egg production.

Hormone imbalance is very closely linked to skin disorders and other diseases. By consuming animal products full of synthetic hormones, as well as the animal's own natural hormones (especially in dairy products, since many dairy farmers keep cows pregnant 300 days a year to increase milk production[10]), you are also interfering with your body's own hormonal balance.

Buying local food is a good idea because the sooner you get it after it's been harvested, the more nutrients it's going to have. It's ideal to consume produce as close to fresh-picked as possible to receive the most benefit from all of those vitamins, minerals, antioxidants, and other nutrients that the skin needs so much.

### The good guys versus the bad guys

Fermented foods—meaning probiotic foods—are particularly beneficial for detoxification. Probiotics are healthy strains of bacteria and microflora. This can be confusing for some people, because in our Western medicine-based society, we are taught that bacteria and other microbes are bad and make us sick. However, we all have bacteria on the skin and in our bodies at all times. Some are harmful (pathogenic), but the majority are beneficial (non-pathogenic) and necessary for proper immune function and digestion.

These friendly flora are the good guys. They run around in our gastrointestinal tracts keeping harmful bacteria (the bad guys) under control and their population in check. Unfortunately, because we are regularly exposed to such a heavy toxic load due to our diets and lifestyles, more harmful bacteria invade and overpower the good guys. They also fortify the existing bad guys and make them stronger (Candida is a very good example of this).

Furthermore, we've become too accustomed to using antibacterial soaps, hand sanitizers, body washes, surface and air sprays, and antibiotic drugs. These materials disrupt our body's balance of good bacteria and harmful bacteria in many ways. Obviously, the theory is that these agents kill only the harmful bacteria. If that were the case, though, then why do so many people get yeast infections and diarrhea when they are taking antibiotics? To be clear, I'm not telling anyone not to take antibiotics if prescribed by a qualified health practitioner. I'm providing information that suggests these medicines and hygiene products may not be needed nearly as much as they are currently used.

The fact is, antibiotics cannot decipher which bacteria are "good" and which are "bad"; they just kill them all. Taking a course of antibiotics is like launching a nuclear attack on your body—all bacteria and microflora, good and bad, die—and guess who begins to repopulate first? The bad guys. The army can't rise from the dead, and bad guys will still find their way in the same way they did before. This is why you need to send in more troops by eating probiotic-rich foods.

Another way antibiotics and antibacterial agents disrupt the inner ecosystem is by creating drug-resistant strains because the existing bacteria, yeasts, and viruses become immune to them. Remember, these microbes want to survive, and they multiply quickly. When they're threatened, they mutate in order to adapt, which create stronger, more resistant strains that are harder for our bodies (as well as antibiotics) to fight off. It keeps the immune system in constant action, which is very stressful for the body. This may be one reason for the rise of autoimmune disease that affects a larger population more than ever before.

**The Candida conundrum**

To further complicate the issue, let me introduce you to Candida albicans. Candida albicans is a particularly resistant strain of yeast that naturally occurs in various parts of the body. Yeast is a spore and spores are the most resistant organisms on Earth. They remind me of cockroaches—you know how people say cockroaches would likely be the only species to survive a nuclear attack? Make that cockroaches and Candida. Candida's main job in the body is to decompose tissue after we die. In an ideally healthy body, the numbers of Candida albicans would be controlled by healthy intestinal microflora so they wouldn't have a chance to do any damage until they were actually needed—at which point we wouldn't care because we'd be gone. However, most modern Western diets are very high in toxins and other substances that Candida feeds on—sugar, alcohol, and bread for example. Candida also feeds on already decomposing material, which unfortunately, many people have in abundance in their digestive tracts from eating high amounts of meat and other foods that have not been properly digested. Under-digested meats begin to rot, which is like an all-you-can-eat buffet for the yeast. They feed, they grow even stronger, and they multiply rapidly.

You might be wondering what this has to do with the skin. I didn't make the connection until I attended a workshop at a spa show called, "Candida Screening and Consultation, " presented by Linda T. Nelson, N.D., Ph.D.[11] When I initially saw the workshop title, I have to admit it did not interest me at all. It actually grossed me out. I thought to myself, "Yeast? Ew. What does that have to do with skincare?" However, several colleagues told me the class was very interesting and I had already heard about yeast overgrowth from a family member who had become very ill from it, so I decided to attend.

After taking the class and doing further research, I found that nearly every chronic condition, mental and physical, can be traced back to Candida overgrowth; not just in women, but also in men. These symptoms include migraines, obesity, multiple sclerosis, lupus, depression, endometriosis, athlete's foot, miscarriages, hypothyroidism, acne, eczema, psoriasis, rosacea, and many more. I was shocked and wanted to learn more, especially since I had several of those conditions at the time I took the class: I was overweight; had acne, experienced bouts of depression, and had just been diagnosed with subclinical hypothyroidism. When I found out Dr. Nelson's company was offering a Candida detoxification certification course in my area shortly after the show, I promptly signed up.

Most people only associate Candida, or yeast, with vaginal yeast infections or thrush. Unfortunately, these infections are just the tip of the iceberg, and are actually symptoms of a much larger, systemic problem. Candida overgrowth is very detrimental to the entire body. It attacks the whole immune system and can contribute to serious, chronic ailments, as well as skin disorders.

In the meantime, I asked my primary care doctor about Candida overgrowth in general. She implied that controlling yeast in the body and eliminating foods that feed yeast to treat chronic illnesses are the beliefs of new-age space cadets who have probably smoked too much wacky tabacky. I was highly insulted; especially since I already knew that other forms of healing (which existed thousands of years before Western medicine) consider Candida overgrowth to be a major cause of disease. However, my doctor was an MD, not a holistic practitioner, naturopathic doctor, or nutritionist. It just wasn't an idea in her realm of expertise.

**Candida needs to be treated holistically.**

One question I had when I was learning about all of this was, "What about those medications for yeast infections?" Remember how I mentioned that medications like antibiotics are like nuclear warheads in your body? And what two organisms would be the only ones to survive a nuclear attack? Cockroaches and Candida.

Candida cannot be effectively treated with traditional antifungals and antibiotics. While these options may offer relief in the short-term, they are actually doing more damage to the body in the long-term.

In her book, *Living Symptom-Free: Fibromyalgia & Candida*, Dr. Nelson states: "Drugs that specifically address fungus or Candida destroy some of the yeast. The yeasts that are not affected by the drugs begin to colonize in vast numbers and become more and more drug-resistant. As yeast multiplies in its stronger state, they produce toxins that attack the body's defense (immune system). These same drugs also destroy the friendly bacteria or flora in the body so that there is no defense against the new, stronger fungus."[12]

**The only way to kill a drug-resistant organism is to starve it.**

If you have any of the symptoms of Candida overgrowth, look at your diet.

Candida overgrowth can only be managed by reducing and/or eliminating yeast-containing foods, as well as foods that feed or grow yeast. It's also important to add more probiotic-rich foods and supplements into your diet to replace the "good" bacteria and flora that was destroyed by the yeast, and help eliminate the remaining harmful bacteria and flora. Doing a cleanse or structured detox is very beneficial because the dead yeast spores will accumulate as toxins. In addition to diet, certain herbs, spices, and essential oils will help the body dislodge the toxins and eliminate them.

There are many detoxification programs available that are specific to Candida cleansing. Like any other cleanse, I only recommend following these programs under the guidance of a qualified and knowledgeable health professional trained in different cleansing/detoxification methods. This way, your cleanse will be tailored to your specific needs and can be adjusted along the way based on your progress throughout the program. There are so many pre-packaged cleanses out there it's hard to know which one is best for you, or if it is even safe. No single cleanse is right for everyone, because everyone's constitution and needs are different.

**You might be wondering why the body needs help detoxifying itself.**

The human body was very intelligently designed. It was made to carry out its essential functions as needed to keep it running properly. It shouldn't need techniques, tools, products, and spa treatments to work as it should.

Visualize a perfect, pristine place. Maybe it's a tropical paradise far from civilization and industry. It has an abundance of clean, fresh water, pure air, and a large variety of naturally growing, whole, local, seasonal, unprocessed foods free of pesticides, steroids, hormones, antibiotics, fillers, preservatives, and other artificial additives. We never have to work, we spend all day in a stress-free land surrounded by happy people we love, and we get ample physical activity and rest. Our bodies easily digest our fresh foods and easily fight off any rare threat of disease. Does this ideal situation exist anywhere on our planet today? Sadly, no.

If you are someone who regularly eats all natural, organic, balanced meals;

gets adequate hydration, rest, and exercise; avoids unhealthy substances and lifestyle choices; and takes great care of yourself all around, then you're already doing the right things.  You probably have great skin too, which is visible evidence of the overall health of your body. Most of us, though, need a little help.

It's not the body's fault. It knows what it was designed to do. However, the mind and bad habits often prevent the body from doing what it was meant to do. So, if we cleanse the body, inside and out, we can start working with it instead of against it.

**A detox, or a "cleanse" is just what it sounds like.**

It is a regimen that cleanses the body of toxins and other unwanted matter from the inside out. There are as many different ways to cleanse as there are different types of toxins. Some are powders that can be mixed into beverages while others are herbs in pill or tea forms. There are cleanses that rely on juicing alone or eating one type of food for long periods of time; and some require eliminating certain foods from the diet for a period of time, then reintroducing them later on. Other cleanses rely on certain foods alone with no supplements or other tools. There are also different cleanses to cleanse different organs: the liver, the colon, the intestines, the pancreas, even the skin.

Cleanses also typically involve exercise (toxins are excreted through sweat) and meditation or spiritual practice (to release stress and other emotional toxins that can be just as damaging as physical toxins).

Remember that the follicles of the skin must be clear and unblocked so that they can perform their jobs of secretion and excretion—in this case, I am referring more to the excretion of toxins through the sweat. One great way to promote this action is to incorporate daily dry brushing of the body into your regimen.

# Dry Brushing[13]

The function of sweating is crucial to the body's natural detoxification process. In fact, the skin is responsible for excreting approximately one pound of waste products per day primarily through the sweat glands, which accounts for one-quarter of the body's total daily waste.

Malfunctioning sweat glands can also cause blockages in the lymphatic system, which can lead to an unhealthy buildup of lymph (bodily fluid responsible for collecting and transporting waste products to detoxification organs for elimination), which can cause swelling in the limbs and joints. It also adds unnecessary stress to the body, making it work harder to eliminate the additional waste, which forces it into a state of imbalance.

It may be hard to imagine that perspiration serves such an important function. Many people simply associate it with that salty, unpleasant moisture that we have to wipe away after exercise or on hot days. However, "chemical analysis of sweat shows that it has almost the same constituents as urine."[14] You don't want that trapped in your body or skin. Like urine and other forms of excrement, better out than in.

**Dry brushing keeps sweat glands clear and promotes healthy perspiration in addition to these other benefits:**

- Increases blood circulation
- Stimulates and cleanses the lymphatic system
- Helps break up and remove toxic build-up in the fat cells, which reduces cellulite
- Improves the overall appearance of the skin by softening, tightening, and toning it
- Helps improve muscle tone
- Fortifies the immune system
- Removes dead skin cells, dirt, built-up oils, and other debris from the surface of the skin to keep the sweat and oil glands functioning properly. This also helps to prevent dry skin, and does not compromise the skin's natural barrier (unless you overdo it).
- Strengthens the skin's immune system, which helps strengthen the body's immune system

I realize all of this information about detoxification can be overwhelming, and you might be wondering where to start. **The Holistically Haute™ Dry Brushing and Salt Bath Ritual** is an inexpensive ritual I've developed that can be done once a week, in the comfort of your own home.

## How Do I Get Started?

First, go to your local health food/natural product store or apothecary and purchase a brush made of natural bristles (synthetics are usually meant for scrubbing dishes or bathroom surfaces and are too harsh for the skin). Bristles can be sourced from certain animals (wild boar, goat), or plants (palms, sisal or other grasses, loofah) depending on your preference. They come in various sizes and fiber strengths. Choose a gentle brush, preferably with a long handle for hard-to-reach areas.

The majority of the body can be dry brushed (but never the face), typically once a day before showering (twice if you are sick, stressed, feel bloated or otherwise sluggish). The procedure is called dry brushing because the skin and brush must be dry. I shouldn't have to say this, but I will just to avoid any confusion: you have to be naked for this.

It is very important to gently, but firmly, brush the entire body **from the tips of the extremities towards the core**. On the core itself, you can brush sideways or in a gentle, circular motion (to massage the organs), but always inward towards your center.

After dry brushing, tap the brush over the trash to remove the dead skin cells from the brush, and then put it away. Don't wash it...that will cause bacteria or fungi to grow in the brush, and it will have to be thrown out. Once you put it away, jump into the shower. There are differing opinions on whether a hot or cool shower is best. Some people even say to alternate hot and cold temperatures while in the shower. I say just take a shower that is a comfortable temperature for you, but never too hot.

## The Holistically Haute™ Dry Brushing and Salt Bath Ritual

This should be done close to bedtime, because you'll want to go to sleep when you are done.

1. **Perform a thorough dry brushing.** This begins the detoxification process of the skin as well as the internal organs and fluids.

2. **Add a cup or two of pink Himalayan or Dead Sea salt** (Epsom or Celtic Sea salt if you don't have the others—these are available at most health food stores and online), or a high-quality, pre-mixed, salt-based, detox bath soak to a full tub of very warm, but not hot, water. Add several drops of your favorite essential oil. Lavender is my preference for fragrance, but rosemary and helichrysm are the best for helping the salts pull toxins out through the skin. The water should be very warm—you should be able to submerge yourself without discomfort from excess heat. Relax and clear your mind. This is not the time to think about your business meeting tomorrow, the kids, or financial worries. Be quiet and peaceful: just be. If you meditate, practice visualization, or any other mental relaxation techniques, this would be the perfect time and place.

3. **Stay in the bath for no more than 20 minutes.** Get out, let the water drain out, and gently towel off. Go straight into a cool shower but not too cold as this will shock the body. Use a good washcloth or gentle scrubbing gloves to remove any excess salt and toxins from the skin. Afterwards, it is nice to apply a light, all-natural moisturizer. Once you've finished the ritual, get thee to bed and dream sweet dreams. Your mind, spirit, and body should be totally relaxed, clear, and at peace, leading to an amazing night of sleep.

# Chapter 7: How What You Eat Affects Your Appearance

Now we know that the amount of toxins built up in our bodies determines not only our internal health, but also the health and appearance of our skin. We also know how important it is to keep Candida and other "bad guys" in our GI tract in check by bringing in more "good guys"— probiotics. Now, it's important to understand how to do this on a regular basis—not just by doing one big cleanse or detox program. Remember, the more we can do to help the body regularly perform its own detoxification through diet and lifestyle, the healthier, stronger, and yes—more attractive—we'll be. Also, keep in mind that built up toxins negatively affect emotions, so when we're trying to heal from any condition, we need to make sure all paths are clear for physical and emotional healing.

When we eat healthy, whole foods we produce healthier cells and take in fewer toxins. The foods we eat also have a strong effect on our hormones, which play an important role in the health of our skin. There is a very strong connection between certain foods that trigger higher levels of hormones and others that can actually lower those levels. Making dietary changes can help regulate hormonal imbalances, which will reduce the possibility of a hormonal skin reaction.

There are so many myths about what foods cause acne and debates about whether foods even have the ability to cause acne or not. If you've gotten this far, I think you probably know by now that not only can foods cause or worsen acne, rosacea, and other skin conditions, they also have the ability to heal them.

When it comes to diet and nutrition, there's no one particular diet or theory that will produce positive results in every person. The reason is because we were all born with different physical, emotional, and behavioral traits or constitutions. In addition, we all come from different ethnic backgrounds. We were raised eating different kinds of food and have different values, triggers, and emotional connections to food. We also lead different lifestyles and have access to different kinds of foods depending on where we live and work.

The United States is often referred to as a "melting pot," because people from all around the world come here to live and work. How could one diet possibly suit every need of every individual person in such a diverse population?

There is also a lot of conflicting "evidence" about what the human body was designed to eat and what the earliest humans actually ate. Some insist that anthropological evidence proves that humans aren't omnivores but were always meant to be herbivores due to the shape of the teeth, the length of the GI tract, and the fact that we're not built with the strength or speed of other meat-eating animals. There are also high-protein diet advocates, like those who favor the Paleo/Caveman diet and believe that early humans were not only omnivores, but leaned more toward being carnivores because they needed high amounts of protein, saturated fat, and essential fatty acids to survive their physically demanding lifestyles. These proponents claim that once humans began consuming grains, their health began to deteriorate. People who subscribe to the raw food theory take this one step further, believing that once humans learned to cook at all is when their health began to deteriorate. **The conundrum with all these theories is that they all have proof that their way is the absolute truth!**

Personally, I believe human beings are omnivores, but I think we should eat more plants than animals. The majority of research across different cultures seems to indicate that cultures who consume more plant foods and less animal foods live longer, healthier lives. Raw foods should be incorporated into our diets, but I don't think that eating cooked food will necessarily make people sick. Of course, there are correct and incorrect ways to cook food—obviously, it's important to make sure food is prepared at the correct temperature using proper methods—but I don't think that human beings would have figured out how to boil water and cook food if we weren't meant to cook food.

The same applies to eating grains. So many diets paint carbohydrates as the enemy—that they make you fat. Many, however, don't teach dieters which ones actually do. There are different types of carbs—whole grains, seed-like grains and grasses (wheat, oats, quinoa, brown rice, wild rice, millet, buckwheat), and refined grains (pasta, bread, white rice, flour). These refined grains have been stripped of their bran and germ—both of which contain fiber, enzymes, and other nutrients necessary for the body to properly recognize, digest, and absorb the food. What's left is a white, mushy substance that the body interprets and digests as sugar. In terms of whole grains, some people tolerate all of them—others tolerate none of them—but most people tolerate and benefit from some of them. Which ones? You'll have to try them and see how your body likes them.

It's really easy to be seduced by charismatic personalities who have a band of celebrity testimonials claiming that their diet is the only way to health. While there's a lot of conflicting information out there, there are also some common threads. Overall, most dietary theories agree that we should be eating high-quality, fresh foods. One of my favorite quotes that answers the question of "What should I eat?" comes from Michael Pollan's book, *In Defense of Food: An Eater's Manifesto*: "Eat food. Not too much. Mostly plants."[15] Simple. Done.

**There are some foods that are known to be beneficial and protective of the skin.**

These foods hydrate, provide nourishment, and prevent damage so that the cells that come to the surface are healthy and strong. These foods also help facilitate the body's continuous detoxification process and don't feed or strengthen the "bad guys" or promote Candida overgrowth.

On the flip side, there are several foods and substances that are common triggers for skin conditions. These substances create an acidic environment, disrupt digestion, feed Candida, and create toxins that attack the "good guys" and strengthen the harmful bacteria and yeasts, and promote inflammation and free radical damage at a cellular level. The biggest problem is that most people consume these foods and substances on a regular basis, and worse, have been taught that many of them are healthy. What are they?

**The "Skin Trigger Trifecta"**

Warning: this is where I tend to lose people, so stick with me. The three foods/substances—AKA the "Skin Trigger Trifecta"—that are known culprits for skin conditions such as acne, eczema, rosacea, psoriasis, keratosis pilaris, melasma, seborrhea, and others are:

- Refined Sugar
- Gluten
- Dairy—especially pasteurized dairy

Aagh! It's crazy, right? Don't close the book, keep reading!

People often ask me, "If I can't eat that, that, and that, then what the heck can I eat?" Then they freak out because they think I'm not going to let them eat anything and that they're going to starve to death. They begin to weigh out the situation and consider what's more important: eating pizza and ice cream or clearing up their skin?

When I first learned that the Trifecta was possibly the culprit behind my own skin condition and inability to lose weight, I thought never having ice cream, pizza, or pasta again was like getting the life sucked out of me. These were three of my biggest culinary pleasures in life—plus I've got Italian blood running through these veins. Wouldn't cutting out bread, pasta, mozzarella, and parmesan cheeses make me a bad Italian? What would I eat at family functions? And God forbid I ever go back to Italy— I'd be completely screwed (of course, the rational thought of eating a modified, Mediterranean diet never crossed my mind). I also had a sweet tooth with a mind of its own. I still enjoy sweets now and then, but the cravings are few and far between compared to how they used to be and I choose my sweets much more carefully now.

In my totally freaked out thought process, I also remembered that life-changing conversation with my sister when she told me that since I was not getting the results I wanted with my current choices, then clearly I was not doing enough and I was not making the right choices for my body. It's just like the definition of insanity: "doing the same thing over and over again and expecting different results."[16] I strongly disliked what I knew was coming—eliminating the Trifecta to see if it was truly the reason behind my misery. But I already knew it was true—the more I read about the Trifecta, holistic skincare, nutrition, and Candida, the guiltier I felt every time I reached for a cookie or slice of pizza.

This was a different kind of guilt too, because I was making those choices with the full knowledge that by doing so, I was likely making my condition worse and reducing my chances of ever getting better. Self-sabotage is a common defense mechanism, and not just in terms of food.

**To me, this created a new definition of insanity:** Doing the same thing over and over again *having full knowledge of the likely outcome* and STILL expecting different results—this is also known as DENIAL.

I finally realized how ridiculous that was and allowed myself to step into the unknown world of food that didn't include dairy, sugar, or gluten. I'm not going to say it was easy. In fact, it really sucked. I hated having to explain myself at family functions, feeling so limited when ordering at restaurants, and I really hated walking past my favorite indulgences at the grocery store knowing I couldn't have them.

But you know what? It got better, and sooner rather than later. My weight began to melt off and my skin cleared up completely within weeks. I also had more energy, better moods, and clearer thoughts. I felt that the funky haze that I had been in (which I had previously associated with being a mom of a toddler and a baby) had finally lifted and I began to feel like myself again. I was also starting to feel really proud of myself I began to look at my body with a new sense of awe because, for the first time in years, it was actually doing what it was designed to do. I began to respect and love it, and I also found a new love for my spiritual and emotional self because I had the intelligence, the strength, and the resolve to make this tough decision. I felt so great, I wanted more.

## Why does the Trifecta cause skin conditions?

Sugar, dairy, and gluten are hard to digest for various reasons—one of which is they are too prevalent in our food supply. In most other cultures, they either are not part of traditional diets, or they are eaten in moderation. They also feed Candida.

Gluten is a protein found in wheat, barley, corn, and other whole grains and seeds. It's actually really easy to go gluten-free when you are eating real, whole foods. While some whole grains and seeds naturally contain gluten, many don't (quinoa, amaranth, millet, buckwheat, rice, etc.). Processed and packaged foods contain large amounts of gluten because it's a cheap way for manufacturers to meet the FDA's protein requirements on food labels. It's also an excellent binder, which is why flour is used to thicken sauces, dressings, and hold together breaded or fried foods and baked goods. So many ingredients contain gluten, that unless you carry a lengthy list to the store and crosscheck every single label, you'll be grocery shopping for hours. This is also the case at restaurants, unless they have a gluten-free menu. Many sauces and dressings (even on seemingly healthy salads) contain gluten.

Different forms of refined sugar are also highly abundant in processed, packaged, and restaurant foods. Why? To make foods taste better so people want them more. Sugar is also extremely addictive—in fact, it's more addictive than many illicit drugs.

### What's the Most Addictive Drug? The Answer Might Surprise You.[17]

Before I began learning about holistic skincare and nutrition, I was aware that artificial sweeteners were associated with many different health risks and that some were even potential carcinogens. I thought that it would be better to just use real sugar, but in moderation. After awhile, my own sugar cravings became out of control, and I'm sure it was a significant contributing factor in my own weight gain. There's a reason for that: refined sugar (white table sugar) is not "real" sugar after all. It's not a whole food, and has been heavily processed, therefore stripped of any nutritional value that would've helped the body digest it properly. It's an addictive, toxic substance and should be avoided... it really is nothing that resembles actual food at all. Even raw sugar has been heavily processed. These sugars are closer in molecular structure to illicit drugs and are even more addictive.

It's possible to satisfy a sweet tooth without consuming processed sugar. There are many sugars existing in whole food forms found in nature, some of which cause less of a glycemic reaction than others. Pure maple syrup, pure raw coconut nectar (sap from the coconut palm tree), and raw honey are whole foods containing natural sugars (fructose). Although they will cause blood sugar levels to rise, these foods are healthier choices overall because they retain their vitamins, minerals, antioxidants, enzymes, and other beneficial nutrients, which will slow down the digestive process and glycemic reaction. These foods are safe to consume in moderation in place of white table sugar.

When you're in the beginning stages of healing, even certain fruits and natural sugars should be avoided until the condition has resolved. These can be reintroduced slowly after. Another natural option for sweet flavoring is pure stevia (a South American herb) extract or powdered dried stevia. Stevia doesn't contain any sugar and won't produce a glycemic reaction or exacerbate Candida overgrowth or skin conditions.

Dairy—meaning products made from cow's milk —is not easily digested by humans, especially pasteurized dairy. Cow's milk and human mother's milk are very different in chemical structure. When we're babies, we naturally produce an enzyme (lactase) that's meant to properly break down breastmilk. As we grow older, we no longer produce this enzyme because our bodies begin to require nutrients from other whole foods. Therefore, our bodies can no longer properly digest human milk, much less milk or products processed from cow's milk that contains enzymes and proteins the body may not even recognize or know how to digest.

This is a controversial topic, and the reason is largely due to politics, not nutrition. It's important to note that the majority of the problem with dairy products is that they are made from pasteurized milk. This means the milk or dairy products have been heated to extremely high temperatures to kill any pathogenic bacteria or viruses. The problem with that is similar to the problem with antibiotics—the process also kills any nutritional benefits that the milk may have had. Raw milk from grass-fed cows contains high-quality fats, as well as beneficial bacteria and enzymes necessary for proper digestion. It's a whole, complete food that some people are able to tolerate and digest quite well. Raw milk, however, isn't recommended by the USDA and many state governments have banned its distribution claiming health risks due to potential contamination. However, the majority of all milk recalls have been for pasteurized milk.

Here's the thing about pasteurization—yes it kills germs, but it only kills them at a certain point in the process. It doesn't provide any immunity to subsequent contamination during processing and handling. Properly handled raw milk still contains its own little army of healthy bacteria, so it actually has a better chance of avoiding contamination than pasteurized milk.

While raw milk is a healthier option than pasteurized milk, it's produced when a cow's hormone levels are high, and those hormones are excreted in the milk. It's also mucus-forming, and if it's not digested properly (which it won't be in most cases), it will begin to putrefy and produce toxins that will attack the body's healthy bacteria and feed Candida. While fermented milk products like kefir and yogurt are slightly easier to digest and do introduce some good bacteria into the equation, I still believe these products should be limited or avoided completely, especially for people with digestive issues and/or skin conditions.

I know what you're thinking: dairy is a food group! Kids are taught in school and parents are taught by pediatricians that milk is necessary for good bone health because of the calcium and vitamin D. The truth is that milk is only a good source of calcium and vitamin D if it is unpasteurized, whole milk processed from grass-fed, pasture-raised cows. Conventionally raised cows live indoors in horrible conditions with little-to-no exposure to sunlight. Their bodies aren't able to produce any Vitamin D naturally. Calcium needs two things to be absorbed: fat and Vitamin D. The majority of milk products available in our food supply today are low-fat or skim, and come from factory-raised cows.

Unfortunately, politics are the reason for this whole belief that dairy products are healthy—the same can be said for gluten. Think about the USDA food pyramids and even the newer My Plate versions (these, thankfully, place less focus on dairy and more focus on fresh fruits and vegetables). According to these images (that are being taught to children), pepperoni pizza would be considered a healthy food. It contains bread (carbohydrate), vegetables (tomato sauce), dairy (mozzarella), protein (pepperoni), and fat (nasty grease that drips down from melted mozzarella and pepperoni). See? It contains all food groups, therefore it is a complete meal according to the USDA. Does anyone else see a problem with that? Clearly there's a huge disconnect between what's actually healthy vs. what's taught to be healthy.

> For more on food and American politics, visit Marion Nestle's website www.foodpolitics.com. For more about raw vs. pasteurized dairy, visit www.realmilk.com.

There are other foods and substances besides the Trifecta that may trigger skin conditions in some people who have an underlying food sensitivity, intolerance, or allergy. Tree nuts, peanuts, and nightshade vegetables are some potential triggers.

Alcohol is a very common trigger for acne as well as rosacea. I know you probably needed a drink after reading about the Trifecta. I can't tell you how much alcohol is appropriate for you—that has several variables, and obviously, certain physical and emotional health concerns contraindicate drinking any alcohol at all. If you tend to become flushed, experience digestive issues, break out, or notice visible capillaries in the corners of your nose or on your cheeks after consuming alcohol, your body may be telling you to stop.

### How can I eliminate these food triggers without having massive cravings?

This is one of the most common questions people ask when I talk about "cleaning up the diet" to improve skin. I also believe that this concern is one of the main reasons why people have such a tough time getting motivated to eat healthier. No one likes to be told they can't have something—especially when raised to believe it was healthy! Society also teaches us that sugar is a reward. As a parent, I find it very frustrating that my kids' teachers reward them with candy and treats for a job well done or bribe them by using small candies for them to sort, group, or count during a math exercise. If they do it correctly they get to eat the candy.

Many people have also been conditioned to believe that sugar equals love and security. How many grandparents give children cookies or bring their famous pie to the holiday party and everyone eats it because they love Grandma and Grandma loves them? It's hard to be told that these delicious treats packed with Vitamin L (Love) could be causing our skin and health problems.

I often encourage people to eat more good food as they eliminate harmful foods because the body then begins to crave healthy food. There are also substitutions that may help ease cravings. When you cut out sugar from candy or coffee, for example, there are natural sugars that you can add to your diet like fruit, and small amounts of raw honey, and maple syrup. There are some people that do just fine going "cold turkey" with an elimination diet. Others prefer to go slowly and eliminate one thing at a time, adjusting slowly. Everybody is different. Understand that when you have a craving for "bad" foods, they often aren't real cravings. It's better to learn more about what's causing the craving than just to give into it. This does require some mindfulness, which can take practice.

**Now, the good news!**

We've talked about food groups to leave out of your diet if you have a skin condition. Let's focus on foods you can enjoy regularly to help you have gorgeous skin. Here is my list of food groups for **Holistically Haute™ and Healthy Skin:**

- Water
- Essential fatty acids
- Fresh and colorful fruits and vegetables
- Whole grains
- Greens
- Proteins

**Let's start with water.**

On average, the human body is comprised of 50% to 80% water. Every cell, tissue, organ, and system of the body contains water. Our bodies also regularly lose a large amount of water due to perspiration, elimination, and trans-epidermal water loss (TEWL), which is water lost as it evaporates from the skin. The body's hydration must be replenished by water constantly throughout the day to function properly. If you don't drink enough water, your cells can't regenerate, toxins can't be eliminated, food can't be properly digested, your body temperature can't be regulated, and your metabolism slows down.

*"If you don't replenish yourself with water, you will become dehydrated inside and outside. If there are extreme weather conditions, or if you sweat more due to regular exercise, the body loses even more water, so you need to consume even more to make up for it. The skin is a telltale sign of what's going on inside the body. If the body is dehydrated, the skin will show it. It will appear lackluster, possibly flaky and tight, fine lines and wrinkles will be more evident, and it will become irritated more easily. On the body, the skin will be flaky and may even crack. This is not the same as having a chronic dry skin condition. This dehydration is a result of not drinking enough water."*[18]

Adequate hydration is also very important to maintain the skin's cell turnover rate. This is the amount of time it takes for the plump new skin cells (keratinocytes) generated in the deeper layers of the skin to rise to the surface (flattening on the way up), where they protect the fragile new cells being formed in the deeper layers. These "dead" cells stay at the surface long enough for new ones to rise up underneath, at which point they naturally slough off. Water is the driving force behind this entire process.

The cells need enough water to be healthy in the first place. Secondly, there are enzymes on the surface of the epidermis that help the cells shed when the time is right. Water serves as the catalyst to activate these enzymes. Remember earlier when we talked about how so many women go to the spa for exfoliating treatments to speed their skin's cell turnover rate? It's true that the cell turnover rate naturally slows as we age, but dehydration slows it down even more. Without adequate hydration, those enzymes won't activate to shed the old cells. This signals the deeper layers of the skin to slow down production of new cells. So, instead of going to the spa to sand off or peel off those dead cells, try giving your body the water it needs so it can do the job for you (free of charge).

Most people have heard that they need to drink more water, but many aren't sure how much they need. Is it 8 glasses a day? How big are those glasses? Should I drink water with meals? What if I have a busy day ahead and can't be running to the bathroom every 5 minutes? These are common questions I hear from clients whenever the topic of water consumption comes up. Like the diet, how much water someone needs depends on several factors:

- Weight
- Amount of physical activity
- Climate
- Season
- How many raw foods are in the diet
- Exposure to environmental pollutants like smoke, smog, mold, etc.

**However, this basic hydration formula is a great starting point:**

**Hydration Formula:**

Take your weight and divide that number in half. Drink that number of water in ounces per day. For example, if you weigh 120 pounds, you should drink 60 ounces of water per day.

This may need to be increased depending on the climate, as the weather gets warmer, or if you're working out and sweating a lot. Factor in these variables and increase your intake accordingly.

If your skin is already feeling dry and you feel thirsty, you're likely already dehydrated. The more water you drink, the more hydration your skin will receive. The main message is to not get to the point where you feel thirsty.

That sounds like a lot of water, doesn't it? Is it possible to drink too much water? People with certain health conditions, especially kidney issues, might not be able to have as much. For overall healthy people, this formula is sufficient. If you do have an existing illness or condition, consult with a healthcare professional if water consumption is a concern.

When to drink water is also important. Many people enjoy a beverage while eating meals. However, drinking too much water (or any beverage) while your body is beginning to digest food in the mouth, will dilute your body's digestive enzymes, which could interfere with digestion. It's better to enjoy your water before or after a meal.

I also recommend that people drink the majority of their water first thing in the morning. We wake up in a dehydrated and acidic state, since we're not eating or drinking while we sleep. I drink at least 16 to 32 oz of water first thing in the morning to rehydrate, and neutralize my pH. It also helps me wake up. Early morning water is a good way to encourage healthy morning elimination, especially if you drink it at room temperature or warmer. According to Ayurvedic philosophy, drinking warm water throughout the day helps soften accumulated mucus and toxins so that the body can more easily eliminate them. When you drink a large amount of water first thing in the morning, it takes about an hour to get through your system. If you time it right, you will most likely eliminate it before you leave for work or your morning errands.

It's not a great idea to drink a lot of anything too close to bedtime, because going to bed with a lot of fluids in the system can interfere with quality sleep.

**Let's talk about fat.**

So many people who want to lose weight and be healthy turn to low-fat, no-fat diets, believing that eating fat is the reason behind issues such as weight gain, cellulite, high cholesterol, and cardiovascular diseases. However, just like there are "good" and "bad" carbohydrates, there are also good and bad fats.

The term, "bad" fat mostly refers to saturated fats, trans-fats, and hydrogenated oils. Saturated fats are found in butter, meats, egg yolks, dairy products, as well as smaller amounts in plant foods like coconuts, olives, and avocadoes. Not all saturated fats are bad and not all cause inflammation and illness. In fact, according to renowned osteopathic physician and New York Times Bestselling Author, Dr. Joseph Mercola, consuming the right high-quality saturated fats actually has a protective effect on different parts and functions of the body including[19]:

- Cell membranes
- Liver
- Immune system
- Heart
- Lungs
- Hunger regulation
- Absorption of calcium
- Hormone production and regulation

When choosing products containing saturated fat, look for the highest quality you can find—organic butter, ghee, or beef from grass-fed/pastured cows, eggs from pastured chickens, organic virgin coconut oil, or organic extra virgin olive oil. Saturated fats should still be consumed sparingly, as too much can certainly have adverse effects on health.

However, most of the health problems associated with too much fat in the diet stem from too much trans-fat and hydrogenated fat in the body. Food companies started using these fats in shortening and margarine to replace saturated fats like butter after people began to associate high amounts of saturated fat with health problems. Incidentally, raw milk advocates, like the Weston A. Price Foundation[20], claim that butter and ghee made with raw milk from grass-fed cows doesn't cause these health problems nearly as much as comparable pasteurized products.

These artificial fats are oils that have been chemically altered. They are hydrogenated and then rearranged on a molecular level. During this process, these oils are hardened to more closely resemble butter and make them stable enough to prevent rancidity. This also keeps them intact when cooking or baking at very high temperatures (think deep frying).

This process is also highly industrial, which likely results in a product that contains chemical residues and other hazardous waste products full of free radicals that damage at a cellular level.

Now that several health hazards associated with trans-fats have been widely publicized in medical research and in mainstream media, food manufacturers are beginning to phase them out, replacing them with hydrogenated or otherwise manufactured fats. The problem is that the FDA allows food manufacturers to advertise and list on their packaging that their products contain zero grams of trans-fat. However, the products are allowed to contain up to 500 mg of trans-fats per serving and still be labeled as containing zero grams of trans-fat. If you buy processed and packaged foods, or eat out at restaurants often, it's nearly impossible to know how much trans-fat you are actually consuming. These substances accumulate in the body over time, which produces toxins and causes systemic inflammation, in addition to other health concerns.

**Another "bad" fat is vegetable oil.**

This is a confusing one, because we are taught that vegetables are healthy—so shouldn't vegetable oil be healthy?

The problem is that the "vegetable oil" on store shelves isn't the naturally occurring oil found in plants. Vegetable oil is an altered form of these oils, which creates problems for the body at the cellular level, similar to trans-

and hydrogenated fats. These fats are no longer in their natural state, and the body doesn't know how to handle them. It tries to digest and use them somehow, but we don't have receptors for these foreign substances. The fats end up in places where they don't belong which can wreak havoc on our health. For example, they can deposit in cell membranes where they interfere with that cell's ability to function and reproduce.

**I always like to get the bad news out of the way first, so now let's talk about healthy fats.**

The right types of fats include fats and oils from whole plant foods such as avocadoes, chia seeds, flaxseeds, olives, and coconuts. When purchasing oils made from these foods, look for the words "organic," "cold pressed" (preferably "first cold pressed" in the case of olive oil), and "extra virgin" for olive oil and "virgin" for coconut oil.

Other healthy fats, specifically Omega-3 fatty acids, come from wild-caught salmon, sardines, and anchovies. There are many issues surrounding heavy metal contamination in fish. This is mainly a problem with farmed fish, which is why it is extremely important to know the source of the fish you consume. Smaller fish have fewer contaminants and may be a better choice if you prefer to get your omega-3s from fresh fish rather than fish oil supplements. If you decide to take fish oil supplements, it's important to research how the oil is sourced and processed. Look for one that removes contaminants, doesn't use any additives, and guarantees freshness. If you get a fish oil supplement that smells fishy or funky, it means that it has oxidized or spoiled, at which point it won't do you any good.

Healthy fats are really good for the skin. All that water you're now drinking can evaporate through the skin if it escapes the cells too quickly. Essential fatty acids strengthen the cells and keep the moisture in. They help to build the cells from the inside out. You'll notice if you take fish oil supplements or eat a lot of Omega-3rich foods like salmon, your skin will have a plumper, thicker, more youthful appearance.

Omega-3 fatty acids are also found in grass-fed beef and eggs from pasture-raised chickens. If you prefer a vegan source, you can try chia seeds or flaxseeds, although the essential fatty acids are not as bioavailable from these sources. Walnuts are a great source of Omega-3 fatty acids as well as other nutrients.

**Eat your colors.**

I always tell my kids to look for fresh fruits and vegetables with the brightest colors. Why? Colors equal nutrients—specifically phytonutrients, antioxidants, and vitamins, many of which can't be found in animal products. The darker the color, the higher the antioxidant content. Look for fresh, organic blueberries, raspberries, cranberries, strawberries, pomegranates, açai berries, red and black grapes, goji berries, and blackberries. Citrus fruits like oranges, lemons, grapefruits, and limes are excellent sources of the antioxidant, Vitamin C. In vegetables, look for organic bell peppers, eggplants, beets, tomatoes, sweet potatoes, squash, and carrots. Red and orange vegetables contain carotenoids like beta-carotene and lycopene, which are also powerful antioxidants.

## Fighting Off Free Radicals: Antioxidants[21]

Antioxidants are "substances, such as vitamin C, vitamin E, or beta carotene that counteract the damaging effects of oxidation in a living organism."[22] Oxidation is the chemical reaction that occurs when oxygen is added to a substance. This causes a loss of electrons, which changes the chemical properties of the substance, and transforms it into something different from its original form.

A perfect example is rust. The original substance is an iron statue. Oxygen is added when rain lands on the statue (water is 2 parts oxygen), and the statue begins to rust. The originally dark, shiny metal becomes a dull, reddish-orange color. The process cannot be reversed, and the metal cannot be restored. Rust is physically and chemically a completely different substance than iron.

This same process happens in our bodies. It's tricky, because of course our bodies need oxygen for respiration and cell generation. We can't survive without it. But oxidation still occurs, which leads to free radical formation (due to the loss of electrons). Imagine normally healthy cells and strands of DNA...then imagine them turning to rust. The free radical damage that occurs due to oxidation can potentially alter healthy cells and DNA. This is how mutations happen, and is the cause of most signs of aging, inflammation, and many diseases.

Our bodies naturally produce antioxidants to neutralize the free radical damage that occurs from everyday functions. However, intrinsic factors like stress, poor nutrition, and poor lifestyle choices, and extrinsic factors such as excessive sun or harsh weather exposure and environmental toxins, create many extra free radicals in the body. Our bodies are so bombarded with these free radicals, that they cannot naturally produce enough antioxidants to combat them. Fortunately, many foods contain antioxidants. The body best recognizes and absorbs antioxidants (and all vitamins and minerals) from food sources, rather than supplements, so adding antioxidant-rich foods to your daily diet is the best way to get them.

## Free Radicals 101[23]

To properly explain free radicals, I have to get a little scientific on you. Electrons are negatively charged particles that orbit the nucleus of an atom. They are most stable when they are in pairs. Free radicals are unpaired (single) electrons that are highly unstable, easily excitable, and aggressive. When anything happens to energize or "excite" these single electrons, they steal an electron from a healthy pair in order to stabilize themselves, thus breaking up that pair and leaving that electron single and unstable. This is how mutation happens. The process causes a chain reaction or domino effect, and repeats over and over.

These free radicals, if not neutralized, damage DNA, causing cell mutation and starting the inflammatory process. Here is an example in terms of aging: Cells that the body intended to be healthy pigmentation cells can manifest on the skin as hyperpigmentation ("sun spots" or "age spots"). Cells that were intended to produce healthy proteins like collagen or elastin, instead cause fine lines, wrinkles, or sagging skin. This speeds up the aging process.

**Greens—in a category all their own.**

Greens are, of course, vegetables. However, I place them in their own category because they are that important for healthy skin and a healthy body. I also give them their own category hoping people will give them more attention! Western diets are seriously lacking in greens, and I believe this is one of the reasons for deteriorating health in the U.S.

Dark, leafy greens like romaine lettuce, spinach, collards, chard, dandelion, and mustard greens—as well as cruciferous greens like broccoli, kale, and Brussels sprouts, are some of the most nutrient-dense foods on the planet. They are packed with vitamins, minerals (calcium, anyone?), antioxidants, and even protein. They are also extremely hydrating, contain abundant amounts of fiber and enzymes, and provide nourishment for healthy gut flora—the good guys. Other greens that are great for the skin include watercress, artichokes, and asparagus.

Greens are excellent for aiding the body's natural process of detoxification by enhancing the function of the kidneys, liver, gall bladder, and lungs, as well as reducing inflammation, neutralizing excessive acid, providing hydration, reducing mucus in the body, increasing blood and lymphatic circulation, and boosting the immune system. Greens also help to lift the mood and provide a boost of energy.

Adding more greens into my diet was the first thing I tried that made a dramatic and noticeable difference in my health. I had been suffering with a chronic, unpredictable, and uncomfortable case of irritable bowel syndrome (IBS), as well as chronic fatigue and depression. When I say that having green smoothies for breakfast, as well as adding greens to my other meals throughout the day made me feel like superwoman, I am not exaggerating! I was almost instantly happier and the IBS symptoms disappeared very quickly. I felt much more focused and started to have creative thoughts again ... I also had enough energy to actually act on them. As I stated earlier, I also began to rapidly lose weight without feeling tired or hungry and my skin quickly cleared up.

There are many ways to add more greens to the diet—eating a salad with meals, for instance—but what works best for me is to have a green smoothie for breakfast and for an afternoon snack on a daily basis. Preparing green smoothies is easy. All you need to do is blend up some dark leafy greens and other vegetables like celery, and then add some fresh fruit to make it taste great. I make mine in large batches once a week and either freeze or refrigerate them in glass mason jars so they are always ready to go when I need them.

I'm even going to go so far as to say this: *I think that greens are the key to preventing and curing most diseases.* Of course I now have to point you to the disclaimer in the beginning of this book, having said that—but I really do feel that strongly about the benefits of greens.

**Proteins that benefit the skin**

While the amount of protein human beings actually need to be healthy is yet another of many controversial topics in health and nutrition, protein does specifically benefit the skin.

Protein is very important for any skincare goal. If you want to maintain healthy, youthful-looking, certain proteins will help reinforce the structure and elasticity of the skin. If healing from an inflammatory skin condition like acne or psoriasis is your goal, protein helps promote the body's wound healing functions.

Proteins are found in animal foods like beef, pork, poultry, fish, eggs, and dairy—and if you are an omnivore, it is fine to get your protein in moderate amounts from high-quality sources of these foods (well, except dairy). However, it's very possible to get enough protein from eating a vegetarian or even vegan diet. Proteins are abundant in many plant foods, including dark, leafy and cruciferous greens, whole grains, beans and legumes, nuts, and seeds.

Now I know what you're thinking: how can I eat enough quantity of those foods to get adequate protein? Green smoothies help, but I also add other high-protein foods such as beans and lentils, quinoa, chia, hemp, sunflower, and flaxseeds, walnuts, and almonds to my greens-based stir fry dishes and salads. If you add these foods to your greens, you will have no problem getting your daily protein requirements and staying full until your next meal. I have to admit, I didn't even believe that I could get enough protein from plant foods the first time I heard it. When you think about the amount of greens you'd have to consume to match the amount of protein in a small piece of meat or an egg—not to mention to feel full—it seems overwhelming! How could adding tiny seeds, nuts, and lentils possibly do the trick? I decided to run a little experiment, not just on myself, but on my entire family. I was inspired by a recipe in a vegan cookbook but I didn't have all of the ingredients on hand. While that used to discourage me, I decided to just make substitutions based on what I did have. This is what I came up with:

# Citrus Arugula Salad with Red Quinoa and Mixed Seeds[24]

**Ingredients:**

- 1 cup of pre-soaked/sprouted and rinsed red quinoa
- About 10 oz of baby arugula
- ½ a small red onion, chopped
- 1 tbsp extra virgin olive oil
- ¼ cup rice vinegar or raw apple cider vinegar
- 2 plum tomatoes, chopped or diced
- 2 small cloves of garlic, minced
- Juice from one large orange
- One mandarin orange or clementine, divided with the slices cut in half
- Juice from one lemon
- 2 tbsp raw walnuts, chopped (pre-soaked and dehydrated is best)
- 2 tbsp chia seeds
- 2 tbsp raw and unsalted sunflower seeds
- Himalayan or sea salt with freshly ground multi-colored or black pepper to taste

**Instructions:**

1. Bring 1.5 cups of water to boil on the stove. Add the quinoa. Return to boil, then turn the flame to medium-low, cover the pot, and let the quinoa cook for 15 to 20 minutes. Most of the water should be absorbed, but any excess can be drained. Move the quinoa to a large bowl or baking sheet and refrigerate until cool (this won't take long).

2. In the meantime, chop the onions, garlic, tomato, nuts, and clementine and put them into a large salad bowl. Set aside.

3. In a small mixing bowl, combine the olive oil, citrus juices, vinegar, salt, and pepper for the dressing. Whisk well.

4. Add quinoa and arugula to the veggie/nuts mix, and mix in your dressing. Add the chia and sunflower seeds last, and toss well.

The results? My husband, kids, and I not only loved this salad, we were also completely stuffed. My husband has a big appetite and typically has an extra snack after dinner. I admit that I also sometimes eat a healthy snack if I am working late (or enjoying some downtime catching up with my DVR). That night, and every other night I've made this dish, no one's needed a snack. If I have it for lunch, it sustains me until dinner with no hunger or cravings between meals. So, trust me when I say that you can get all the protein you need, as well as feel satisfied from plant foods!

**How can I fit healthy foods into my limited budget?**

Sadly, junk food and fast food are cheaper than real food, especially organic food. Here are my top strategies for buying healthy foods on a budget:

- **Buy grains, nuts, and legumes in the bulk bins at the health food store.** It's a lot less expensive to buy them that way than it is to buy them pre-packaged or canned.
- **Cook your own food!** Eating in restaurants may be convenient, but it is often more expensive than preparing meals at home. In addition, Sharonah Rapseik, PhD. points out that "We have no idea what goes into restaurant foods. Most take-out and restaurant foods still contain many of the ingredients we should avoid if we are trying to resolve a skin condition—artificial fats, sugar, and salt. Cooking one's own food is key to how fast a condition will start to resolve."
- **Cook extra food so that you have leftovers.** The founder of my nutrition school, The Institute for Integrative Nutrition®[25], Joshua Rosenthal, always says, "Cook once, eat twice." This has been such a meaningful concept for me, especially as a mom who packs her kids' lunches. Instead of processed lunch kits (which look absolutely disgusting, by the way), my kids eat homecooked soups, stews, and stir-fry dishes for lunch at school. This is a great strategy for busy working adults as well. Invest in a high-quality reusable, insulated lunch container and some heat-safe glass storage containers and jars and you're good to go.
- **Grow food when you can!** This is a huge money saver. I can't tell you how many tomatoes I get every summer. Tomatoes, lettuces,

and greens—especially organic ones—are expensive in the store. Of course, what and how much you can grow depends on your climate and the season, but even if you can reduce your food costs for one season of the year, it helps your annual food budget.

- **Use the Environmental Working Group's Shopper's Guide to Pesticides in Produce**[26] at http://www.ewg.org/foodnews/ when you shop. This tells you which foods you absolutely need to buy organic and which ones you can buy conventional without worrying as much about pesticide residue.

### What can I expect when I make a dietary change?

It's different for everyone. Sometimes cravings happen. As the body starts to detoxify, you might experience certain detox symptoms. Go at a pace that feels comfortable for you and fits into your lifestyle. It's helpful to have a coach to help you work through it and support you as you find a plan that will meet your unique needs.

It can be a bit overwhelming at first—just remember that any healthy change is good change. It's progress. Go at a comfortable pace, but don't be afraid to push yourself a little bit out of your comfort zone, because that's when true transformation really happens.

# Chapter 8: Simple Lifestyle Upgrades Can Make a Big Improvement in Your Skin

While your diet has a huge impact on your health inside and out, your lifestyle choices are also a significant factor. It's important to understand that many choices we make in our daily lives can either heal or harm the skin. The most considerable lifestyle factors that affect our toxic load, overall internal health, and skin (inside and outside) are:

- The sun
- Exercise
- Sleep
- Stress
- Exposure to indoor and outdoor pollution
- Alcohol consumption
- Smoking and exposure to secondhand smoke
- Self-care
- Positive and negative influences

**What role does the sun play in the health and appearance of the skin?**

The sun's rays are different wavelengths of radiation. They penetrate the skin at different depths (the epidermis is the outermost layer, the dermis lies beneath, and the subcutaneous fat layer lies beneath the dermis), causing different effects on the cells. For example, the UVA rays are the "tanning" rays, and have long been considered safe since they affect the cells closer to the surface and don't cause burns. These are the rays used in tanning beds and booths, which we now know contribute to skin cancers and premature aging. UVB rays are shorter and more concentrated. They actually penetrate the deeper layers of the skin where they can cause permanent damage and even kill many of the cells.

The sun's rays damage skin cells by either injuring them or causing a permanent mutation in the DNA of the cells. These mutations affect all of the new cells that form subsequently.

I've had the opportunity to interview Tim Turnham, executive director of the Melanoma Research Foundation (MRF), on several occasions. Tim has provided me with excellent information regarding several sun myths, as well as the process of how the rays actually damage the cells. Here's an excerpt from an article I wrote for Technorati[27] regarding the safety of tanning beds:

> "When UVA rays hit the skin, they damage the DNA of the melanocytes (cells found in the deepest layer of the epidermis that produce the body's melanin pigment), which sends them a message and causes them to produce more melanin pigment to protect the skin from additional damage. This emergency response, that so many people consider to be a desirable skin tone, is a tan.
>
> Additionally, David Fisher, MD, PhD, chief of Dermatology at Massachusetts General Hospital/Harvard Medical School states that there is no such thing as a safe tan, since a tan wouldn't exist if DNA damage had not occurred. According to Dr. Fisher, 'Darkening of the skin is caused by damaging DNA. This is the same process by which cancer cells develop…if there's a tan there has to be DNA damage, and with that comes the risk of skin cancer.[28]'"

Causing the melanocytes to darken in defense doesn't just result in a tan or skin cancer. If enough damage is done to the cell, it will remain in a permanent mode of defense and continuously produce more pigment in an isolated area. This is one of the causes of hyperpigmentation—or "sun spots"—which sends many women to the spa to purchase lightening products, peels, microdermabrasion, and laser treatments to make the spots go away. Damaged melanocytes may also permanently darken the entire face—and not in an attractive way. These treatments might be effective for a certain period of time, however, the melanocytes are located in the deepest layer of the epidermis, which most treatments can't reach. They will continue to produce the darker pigment as the cells turn over. Some treatments are aggressive enough to reach this layer (called the stratum germinativum or "basal layer"); however they also increase your risk of additional long-term cell damage.

The sun's rays also harm the cells in the dermis called fibroblasts. When it comes to "anti-aging", fibroblasts are the cells we want to protect the most because they are responsible for producing the precious proteins of youth--collagen and elastin. The damage from the sun's rays actually causes those cells to shut down so they no longer produce these essential proteins.

Collagen gives the skin its structure, thickness, and plumpness. Elastin gives the skin its elasticity and pliability. A great way to see elastin's function in action is to do a pinch test on a young person and then on an older person. Gently pinch the top of a child's hand and you'll notice that the skin snaps back to normal immediately. However, if you pinch the top of an older person's hand, the skin retains the shape of the pinch and takes awhile to return to its normal state.

As we age, the body naturally produces less collagen and elastin. However, damage from the sun's UV rays speeds up this process dramatically, causing visible signs of aging on the skin. Loss of collagen will cause dermal thinning in some areas, while loss of elastin will cause permanent deep wrinkles and sagging (called elastosis). When you add hyperpigmentation into the equation, you end up with uneven pigment, uneven texture, and prematurely lined and wrinkled skin.

While a limited amount of unprotected sun exposure is necessary for the body to produce Vitamin D, the MRF recommends that people take protective measures the majority of the time. Protective clothing should be worn when weather permits and a sunscreen should be used and reapplied as necessary at all other times. Zinc oxide is the sunscreen ingredient I recommend, with titanium dioxide second. These are natural, mineral-based sunscreen ingredients. Chemical or "absorbing" sunscreen ingredients are toxic and produce free radical damage in the body. An important note: just because it's not a warm, sunny day doesn't mean the sun's rays can't be damaging. In the winter when there's snow, the rays can actually bounce off the snow and harm your skin. So, if you're going to be outside shoveling snow, exercising, playing with the kids, or skiing, wear protective clothing and/or sunscreen.

**How does exercise affect my skin?**

Exercise affects the skin directly and indirectly in several ways. Indirectly, exercise raises endorphins, which helps us reduce stress and improve our mood—we frown less and our facial muscles are more relaxed when we're happy. Furthermore, the increased perspiration and physical movement help to stimulate lymphatic flow and drainage, which helps the body dislodge and release toxins. The increased lymphatic flow can also help flush out any pathogenic bacteria or infection that might be present.

Exercise benefits the skin directly by increasing blood circulation, which helps to deliver nutrients to the skin. This improves the overall health of the skin, reduces inflammation, and aids in wound healing if there are any areas of irritation or eruption. It also improves the skin's overall tone, color, and appearance.

## How Does Stress Affect My Skin?[29]

Stress isn't just an emotion we feel. It produces physical reactions in the body. When we're stressed, our brain thinks it's under attack. It responds by jumping into survival mode, and sending out neurotransmitters that activate the hormone cortisol. Cortisol is also known as the "fight-or-flight hormone," or "the stress hormone." When cortisol is released, it takes over the parts of the brain that are normally regulated by hormones that keep us happy, even-tempered, and thinking clearly (the same hormones that are regulated by anti-depressant and anti-anxiety drugs). Instead, the response is similar to that of adrenaline: thoughts are urgent, hyper, and sometimes manic. You may even feel physically and mentally stronger and sharper... as if you're ready for battle.

This isn't always a bad thing, but if the body is constantly forced into this state by chronic stress, it doesn't have time to respond, relax, and return to its normal state. This can result in many health problems, such as depression and other mental illnesses, high blood pressure, compromised immune response, inflammation, hormonal imbalances that can cause problems with blood sugar and body weight, and flare ups of skin disorders like eczema, acne, rosacea, and psoriasis. Any and all of these issues can accelerate the aging process of the skin and even the entire body.

We've already discussed how the health of the digestive tract—the gut—as well as the balance of good guys vs. bad guys affects the skin. However, stress has a direct effect on digestion. When the body is in fight-or-flight mode, it slows or stops many of its functions in order to increase adrenaline, mental sharpness, strength, and speed so we can return to safety. One of these functions is digestion, because under normal conditions, a very large percentage of the body's energy and resources are devoted to digesting and eliminating food. Stress also has a direct effect on the good vs. bad balance of bacteria in the gut, which we know impacts the body's immune system and the skin.

Did you know that stress also has a direct effect on the skin's barrier function as well? A phenomenon called the "hypothalamic-pituitary-adrenal axis" illustrates how "psychological stress disrupts the natural antimicrobial defenses of the epidermis."[30] Remember, the epidermis is the outer layer of the skin and is your first defense against environmental pollutants, the sun's rays, as well as pathogenic bacteria, viruses, and fungi. Compromising its integrity puts the entire body, not just the skin, at risk.

The way in which stress affects the digestive tract and subsequently the skin is referred to as the "gut-brain-skin axis,"[31] and is the subject of ongoing research in both Western medical sciences as well as holistic studies.

According to Dr. Georgia Tetlow, a holistic, integrative medicine physician and Clinical Assistant Professor of Rehabilitation Medicine at Thomas Jefferson Medical College in Philadelphia, "Increased cortisol creates a shift in the balance of friendly and harmful microorganisms in the gut and on the surface of the skin. In the gut, this shift stems from impaired digestion and absorption of nutrients that nourish the skin such as Vitamin B12, the antioxidant alpha lipoic acid, and others. Sustained increased cortisol also disrupts the body's pH, and this disruption of the skin's acid mantle and at the root of the follicles (pores) can be accompanied by hyper-activity of the sebaceous (oil) glands. In addition, deficiencies in key nutrients like zinc and copper speed the skin's aging process by flattening out collagen and elastin fibers in the dermis, which leads to loss of elasticity and dermal thinning."

Cortisol is also directly linked to acne. According to Dr. Ben Johnson, founder and formulator of Osmosis Pur Medical Skincare, "Stress-induced cortisol elevation can cause acne by stimulating the release of toxins currently being stored in their fat.  This overwhelms the system by re-introducing these toxins into the bloodstream, some of which are sent to the skin for disposal. Acne results when the skin attempts to dismantle and remove these toxins.  An acne lesion that takes a long time to heal indicates how potent the toxin is. Rather than focusing on killing the bacteria to heal the lesion, it's more important to find the source of the toxins and remove them. Furthermore, stress cuts off the diffusion of nutrients through the cell walls, which suppresses the immune system and starves the skin. The skin and the body need tools to support the immune system in its effort to heal the skin. Managing stress is one of those tools."

**Positive lifestyle practices effectively reduce stress.**

We live in a stressful world; however, there are some conscious choices you can make that will help reduce the effects of stress on your body:

- Eat healthy, antioxidant-rich foods
- Get enough sleep
- Exercise regularly
- Practice relaxation techniques such a meditation, mindfulness, or yoga
- Keep a regular journal
- Be conscious of breathing deeply and slowly into the belly, rather than inhaling short, shallow breaths into the chest
- Find ways to regularly express creativity—don't be afraid to try something new!

One of the best ways to reduce stress and improve your environment is to get rid of the drama in your life! One way to do this is to unplug regularly, taking frequent breaks from electronic gadgets and the media. We don't need to know every little detail of what goes on in the news, celebrity gossip, or social media.

Also, *deliberately choose to surround yourself with positive people and positive influences* as much as possible. Avoid negativity, which drains your energy and lowers your mood. For example, my husband likes to listen to a talk radio news channel in the car. It plays the same exact information over and over every few minutes and absolutely drives me crazy. It literally makes me want to scream—no offense, Honey, but I don't understand why you listen to this stuff!

Unfortunately, the news rarely focuses on the pleasant, heroic, or positive events that happen in society. The news mainly covers negative events like crimes, accidents, deaths, and natural disasters. I'm not suggesting we ignore the news completely, but repeatedly hearing these negative stories has the ability to alter thought processes. Hearing bad news over and over creates more stress than is necessary. I prefer to get my news by reading headlines on the Internet. If it's something I want to know about, I click to read more. Otherwise, I just skim through and move on. Dwelling on the bad things in society won't help victims of crimes or natural disasters and it won't help your life either.

It's also important to avoid "Negative Nellies." It's OK to excuse yourself from a conversation or hide people's comments on your social media page if their posts bring you down or make you angry. It's even OK to distance yourself from family and friends who haven't traveled on the same path as you have and you find yourself in completely different places. That doesn't mean you end a friendship or disown a family member, but you can choose how often and for how long you will be around that person and under what context.

Choose to focus on topics and surroundings that make you happy, lift your spirits, and spread goodness.

**What does sleep have to do with the skin?**

Sleep is not a luxury, it's a necessity. I'm sure you've been told to go to bed early so that you can "get your beauty sleep." There's truth in that! The body needs sleep to rest and regenerate. It's the only time in a 24-hour day when the body and mind don't physically and emotionally experience stress. When we're awake, we're under constant stress. The only time we're not producing cortisol—the stress hormone—is when we're asleep.

We also don't form as many facial expressions when we're asleep. Remember when your mom used to say, "If you keep making that face it will get stuck like that," or "It takes more muscles to frown than to smile?" While your face won't "get stuck" and the exact number of muscles it takes to frown or smile is undetermined, it is a fact that muscles can be trained. Otherwise bodybuilders would be out of business.

That's one of the theories behind Botox® injections... the clostridium botulinum bacteria paralyze the muscles so they can't "stick" when we frown. By the way, I'd rather try to get more sleep and reduce my stress to prevent expression lines than be injected with botulism any day. But I'm sure you already knew that by now!

I realize that getting enough sleep is a big challenge for most of us— especially those who work late or have children not yet sleeping through the night. But we have to try, nonetheless. A good way to start is to go to bed 15 minutes earlier every night for a week. Then try going to bed 30 minutes earlier the next week and so on. Don't worry...the magic of DVRs, video on-demand, and the online availability of TV shows ensure your shows will be there for you when you have time to watch them. There's no need to schedule your sleep around your shows. If you're up late for other reasons like kids or work, you might have to use creative time management to make sure you get enough sleep.

## How Smoking Affects Your Skin[32]

Most people know that cigarette smoking badly damages the lungs and heart, but it also damages the skin. There's really not much worse you can do for your skin (or health) than smoke.

"Smoker's face" is a term coined in 1985 by Dr. Douglas Model. During his long-term study on the effects of smoking on the skin, he observed physical changes that occurred on the skin of smokers but not on the skin of non-smokers. Dr. Model noted that, "These characteristics were typical of long-term smokers and could be observed regardless of the smoker's age, weight, or degree of sun exposure."[33]

**The physical characteristics of smoker's face are:**

- Dry and dehydrated skin
- Dull, lifeless color
- Prominent lines and wrinkles that occur in places that don't occur on a non-smoker's face. These lines and wrinkles often appear years before they would on a non-smoker's face.
- Loss of elasticity
- Thinning skin
- Areas of mottled discoloration

How and why does smoking cause these physical characteristics of the skin? First and foremost, smoking asphyxiates the skin, meaning that it depletes the skin of oxygen and nutrients. This happens because the toxins, chemicals, and carbon monoxide in cigarette smoke cause the blood vessels to constrict, which slows the circulation of blood and nutrients to the skin. The tiny capillaries located near the skin's surface are not receiving any nutrients, so they respond by dilating (permanently) to allow for more circulation of blood, nutrients, and oxygen.

The army of free radicals unleashed into the body by cigarette smoke causes unfavorable changes to the skin as well as the entire body. Free radicals damage healthy cells and healthy DNA, which can cause them to mutate, or grow abnormally. This causes many problems with the body's functions, which can lead to pre-mature aging and can potentially cause serious diseases like cancer, including squamous cell carcinoma—a cancer of the skin.

Smoking also interferes with the body's production of collagen and elastin, the two protein fibers that keep the skin soft, supple, and firm. The production of these proteins naturally slows with age, but smoking speeds up the process. When the skin is depleted of nutrients and oxygen, it affects the skin's ability to produce new collagen and elastin, as well as "tear down" old and damaged proteins and tissues. If old and damaged tissue is present, new collagen won't form.

## How does drinking alcohol affect the skin?

Consuming small amounts of alcohol in moderation (again, "safe" and "moderate" amounts vary depending on the person), isn't likely to cause a skin problem. However, drinking alcohol regularly and/or excessively negatively affects every organ and system of the body, including the skin.

Drinking excessive amounts of alcohol dumps a large amount of toxins into the body. The liver is the organ primarily responsible for filtering out the body's toxins. Ideally, the liver would adequately filter the alcohol out without causing permanent damage. However, due to stress, lack of sleep, poor digestion, and exposure to toxic chemicals, most people's livers are already overworked. Unloading large amounts of toxins from excessive alcohol is like kicking the liver when it's already down.

The more the liver is overloaded, the more the other detoxifying organs, including the skin, have to overcompensate. This weakens the body's immune system and also reduces circulation to the skin because the blood and lymphatic circulation must first help the liver and other internal detoxifying organs purge the toxins from the alcohol.

The capillaries in the face respond by dilating in an effort to bring more blood and nutrients to the skin (called "vasodilation"), which result in visibly distended capillaries on the skin, commonly in the corners of the nose and on the cheeks. After repeated occurrences, these capillaries can actually dilate permanently, and the condition may eventually progress into rosacea.

According to Dr. Johnson, "Alcohol also unleashes free radicals, which cause liver and protein oxidation. Liver damage also has an effect on hormones, which is linked to melasma . The liver takes a lot of hits from birth to age 30. If the liver is compromised prior to pregnancy, a woman is more likely to develop melasma since her elevated hormones are very taxing to the liver." Aside from hormonal reactions and potentially developing melasma or rosacea, Dr. Johnson notes: "Drinking too much alcohol will interfere with any efforts or protocols to treat or improve a skin condition. In addition to liver damage, the toxins introduced by alcohol also feed Candida, which can lead to overgrowth."

**Think air pollution only affects the lungs? Think again.**

Most people know that breathing in polluted air can have serious adverse effects on the respiratory system. Airborne toxins can also cause cardiovascular distress and liver damage; unbeknownst to many, they also contribute to irritant and inflammatory skin conditions as well as premature aging.

*"Intact and unbroken skin acts as a filter for environmental aggressors such as air pollution, trapping them in the epidermis (outermost*

*layer of the skin that acts as a barrier), which will eventually shed off. However, more and more people have compromised barrier layers because of over-exposure to stressors like the sun, polluted air and water, toxic chemical skin care ingredients, and harsh weather conditions, in addition to intrinsic factors like stress, poor diet, dehydration, smoking, and excessive alcohol consumption. This weakened barrier makes people more susceptible to environmental damage.[34]*

*Air pollutants rob skin cells of oxygen[35] and cause free radical production in the skin. This, in combination with UV radiation, decreases the production of collagen and elastin, causing the skin to thin and lose elasticity. The result is sagging skin, fine lines, and wrinkles.*

*The combination of air pollution and UV radiation also damages melanocytes, the cells responsible for producing melanin pigment. This causes areas of hyperpigmentation on the skin, sometimes in the form of freckles or dark spots, commonly referred to as "age," "sun" or "liver" spots.*

*When toxins and particulates from air pollution become trapped in the epidermis, they can get lodged in the hair follicles (pores) and cause them to clog. This can interfere with the skin's natural ability to slough off dead skin cells and debris, often leading to acne infections such as blackheads, whiteheads, papules, pustules, and acne cysts.*

*Long-term exposure to air pollution can also cause irritant, inflammatory, and allergic skin reactions like rashes, eczema, and blood vessel damage or broken capillaries."*

Though there's not much we can do to reduce the amount of pollution in the air itself, there are certain precautions we can take to reduce our exposure and minimize its effects:

- **Check the local air quality forecast** and take the proper precautions by wearing appropriate protective clothing.

- **Use topical skincare products with antioxidants,** which help to neutralize free radicals that form in the skin before they can enter the body and cause harm.
- **Eat a diet rich in vitamins, antioxidants, and other nutrients.** This will help repair and maintain the skin's barrier layer from the inside out and reduce inflammation and neutralize free radicals.
- **Drink adequate amounts of water.** This will help the skin slough off the dead cells on the surface of the epidermis at a healthy rate and will also help flush out toxins.
- **Use indoor air purifiers and filters;** make sure indoor spaces are properly ventilated.
- **Change air conditioner and heater filters** and clean vents regularly.
- **Decorate with indoor plants** to help filter and oxygenate the air.
- **Open the windows periodically** to let a breeze in and allow for good cross ventilation—even during the winter—especially if there's illness in the home or office.
- **Use all-natural cleaning products** that contain pure essential oils.
- **Avoid synthetic fragrances** in air fresheners, carpet powders, and candles; diffuse pure essential oils instead.
- **Switch your air vent setting to only filter and circulate the air inside the vehicle** when driving through especially polluted areas like construction zones, areas of high traffic, behind a vehicle with dirty emissions, or on salted roads during the winter time. Once you travel to a less polluted area, you can switch the setting back to bringing in air from the outside.

**Practice extreme self-care**

Self-care goes above and beyond a daily regimen. It can be something like making your skincare or hygiene routine a deliberately pleasant experience. It's the act of prioritizing your own care before tending to another. I know to some that might sound selfish, but as I discussed in Chapter 4, it really isn't. It is imperative to make sure your own basic needs are met before you face the day, interact with others, and attempt to give of yourself to others. If you are approaching life with a half-full cup or completely empty cup, then you're just going to drain yourself even more. If your needs are met first, everyone else will benefit.

# Chapter 9: How to Maximize Your Skincare Regimen and Boost Your Hygiene

Now that you know all about how you can improve your skin from the inside out by making healthier choices with diet and lifestyle, it's time to learn about what you can do from the outside in. In this chapter, we'll discuss your skincare regimen, as well as important hygiene issues that make a huge difference in the health of your skin.

**How many products do you have in your regimen?**

Are you someone who likes to keep thing simple with a few essential products, or are you a product junkie like me who loves to try out different things? I admit it...at one point, my bathroom cabinets and shelves resembled a store display rather than just one person's collection! I had a bit of a product addiction—I'd see a flashy advertisement for something new or learn about a new "miracle" ingredient and of course I had to try it for myself—usually without reading the label first. I didn't even care that I still had plenty of product left—after all, a girl's got to have variety right?

Once I became educated about skincare ingredients through my aesthetics training and continuing education, in addition to research I did for articles I wrote on Holistically Haute™, I became a lot more selective. I still had the tendency to "collect" different products, especially after attending spa trade shows and receiving free products to try out and review on my blog—but once I began making my own products and saw how amazing the results were it became very difficult to recommend other products that just didn't work as well as my own.

While I still continue to do some product reviews (hardly any compared to how often I used to do them), I am a lot pickier about the types of products I agree to try and review, especially if there are a lot of ingredients on the labels.

**How on Earth am I supposed to understand all those scientific ingredients on skincare labels?**

Are you a chemist? Me neither. While I've taken some classes and have done a lot of my own research on ingredients in cosmetics—synthetic ones as well as natural ones—I'm not a chemist. And that's OK—you don't need to be a chemist in order to make sound choices in your skincare products, and you certainly don't need to be a chemist in order to make your own at home! I can personally attest to that.

Unless you are a chemist (and even if you are one), there's a pretty good chance that you're not going to recognize the majority of the ingredients on cosmetic labels; especially commercially advertised ones that are primarily man-made and are difficult to pronounce.

**Cosmetic ingredient rule #1: if you can't pronounce it or you don't know what it is it's probably not the best thing for you.**

I've been asked several times if I'd make a cheat sheet for people to take with them when they go to the store so they can read their labels and see if this one's safe, if that one's safe—honestly, there are just too many chemicals to fit onto a cheat sheet. The truth is that there are already many great resources available about cosmetics ingredients. You can buy a cosmetic ingredient dictionary which will tell you all about each ingredient, synthetic or natural. A cosmetic ingredient dictionary will tell you what the ingredient is, what its different uses are, and why it might be necessary in your product. While you might find some information regarding an ingredient's safety, it won't be as comprehensive as other sources such as The Campaign for Safe Cosmetics[2] and The Environmental Working Group's Skin Deep® Cosmetics Database[4].

These resources are great, but think about it. Remember when we were talking about food labels and how no one wants to stand in the aisle at the store for an hour trying to understand every word on every label? The same principle applies to skincare and personal care products. I say just choose products with as few ingredients as possible and make sure you recognize what the majority of them are.

**Cosmetic ingredient rule #2: If the "miracle" ingredient isn't listed in the first five ingredients on the label, don't waste your money.**

What's the deal with all these "miracle" ingredients you see on TV?

It seems like once Oprah gets a hold of it, it's everywhere, right? Like argan oil, for example. There are many ingredients and oils like this that are indigenous to certain remote areas of the world that are very rare and once a celebrity gets a hold of it all of a sudden it's liquid gold and oh my God it's going to heal everything!

Though not all of these miracle ingredients are good, I will say that argan oil is a wonderful ingredient. It's very expensive but it's very beneficial for all skin types and conditions, as well as for anti-aging efforts. But again you have to be careful, depending on who's selling it and how it's marketed. When you see a miracle ingredient on a label or advertisement you have to read the rest of the label and make sure it is listed in that top five.

The first five ingredients make up about 80% of the actual product, so if the first five ingredients are functional ingredients (ingredients that give the product its consistency and help it spread), it won't likely be an effective product. Unfortunately this is the case with the majority of the products on the market. The first ingredient will likely be water, followed by some kind of detergent (example: sodium lauryl sulfate), then maybe a synthetic emollient like mineral oil (a petrochemical), dimethicone (a silicone), or isopropyl isostearate (a synthetic fatty acid), then some kind of polymer or wax (examples: PEG-100 stearate, polyacrylamide or isoparaffin). You might even see a preservative in the top five, like methylparaben, phenoxyethanol, or ethylhexylglycerine. After that you might see something resembling something natural like an extract or oil of some kind of flower, and then maybe some vitamins and some of the bigger cosmetics buzzwords like stem cells or a trendy peptide like Matrixyl® 3000, or a popular antioxidant like Pycnogenol® or resveratrol, and then towards the bottom you will likely encounter the word "fragrance" or "parfum" (these mean the same thing: synthetic fragrance), and then more preservatives.

The example listed above is a completely fictitious label, by the way—and it represents a typical commercially advertised product, not a natural, organic, or handcrafted product. The biggest problem with a formulation like the above example is that even though there are some ingredients that do have the ability to benefit the skin, there are such high percentages of the functional ingredients in the first 5 that the actual therapeutic benefits are either too diluted to be able to make a difference; or there are too many emollient (oils or fats that rest on the surface of the skin and fortify the skin's barrier) and occlusive (ingredients that sit on the surface and don't let anything in or out—these ingredients also interfere with the skin's ability to breathe, secrete oil, and sweat) ingredients in high quantities so that the active, therapeutic ingredients won't even be able to stand a chance of penetrating through the skin's barrier to make any difference on the skin.

### What's the point, you might be wondering?

I hate to sound cynical, but it's all about the bottom line. Active ingredients like plant stem cells, antioxidants, peptides, hyaluronic acid, precious oils like argan oil, and other popular and widely advertised ingredients are very expensive to source. While these large cosmetics manufacturers certainly have money, a large amount of that money goes into multi-million dollar advertising and marketing campaigns often featuring highly paid celebrity spokespeople. Other costs like production, warehousing, transportation, shipping, etc. also affect the bottom line, so this often results in lower priced (and lower quality) ingredients overall, and a practice called "angel dusting." Angel dusting is a bit of a loophole that allows manufacturers to advertise these expensive ingredients on their labels, packaging, and marketing materials as long as they have a certain percentage of that ingredient in the product. That percentage is often too low for the ingredient to actually provide any benefit to the skin.

I have to say I think that's a very deceptive and confusing practice, because it's hard for a consumer to understand why products in several different price ranges all advertise the same active ingredient and claim to have "clinical studies" that prove the product's efficacy. What's important to understand is that while the FDA does require manufacturers to prove a product's safety through a certain degree of testing, the manufacturers don't actually have to substantiate any claims they make in terms of a product's benefits or efficacy. Companies do have to be careful with how they word their claims, because any statement that claims to alter the structure (histology) or function (physiology) of the skin would actually be considered a drug claim; at which point the FDA might intervene and require that the product undergo further testing and procedure to then be labeled as a drug.

There are plenty of functional ingredients that might be listed in the top five ingredients of a natural skincare product like beeswax, water, castile soap, etc.; but the difference is that the majority of natural waxes, oils, butters, and essential oils have their own inherent therapeutic properties. They add to the function of the product but also benefit the skin. Pure aloe vera gel is an excellent example of this. It helps a product spread and also prevents evaporation, which are very functional characteristics. However, aloe vera is also one of the most soothing, hydrating, and anti-inflammatory ingredients found in nature—it also has a temporary tightening effect which might be beneficial in a product marketed as an anti-aging product.

Furthermore, many natural emollients are structurally very similar to human sebum, so even though they help strengthen and protect the skin's barrier, they also have the ability to be recognized by the body and absorb deeper into the epidermis and provide nourishment there. Examples of this are jojoba oil and essential oils. Jojoba oil is a natural plant ester—liquid wax—that closely resembles human sebum and is quickly absorbed by the skin. For this reason, it's an excellent carrier oil for essential oils—meaning it "carries" them into the skin when they are mixed together, rather than blocking them completely like a mineral oil or silicone would do.

Even though natural products contain fewer chemical ingredients, and more ingredients that benefit the skin in some way, angel dusting still does occur. So I'd still recommend that if you're in the market for a product containing a specific ingredient—let's say argan oil—make sure that ingredient is listed in the top five whether it is a chemically-based product or a natural one. I think you know by now that I'd prefer that you choose a natural one.

**Cosmetic ingredient rule #3: Avoid the words "fragrance" and "parfum"— even if they are preceded by the word "natural."**

Here is an excerpt from my article, "Why Synthetic Fragrances Stink"[36], originally published on Blogcritics.org.

> *"The FDA doesn't require companies to individually list all of the ingredients that make up a product's fragrance. They can just say "fragrance", "perfume/parfum", "natural fragrance", and even "unscented." So if you purchase a mango body wash from a store that is not an all natural store, it's very unlikely that you're actually smelling mango, unless the label specifically says otherwise. Instead, you smell a combination of ingredients that make the product smell mango-ish.*
>
> *The problem is that synthetic fragrances are the most likely ingredients in products to cause allergic and irritant reactions, and many of them are toxic. According to the Enviromental Health Association of Nova Scotia's Guide to Less Toxic Products, 'in 1989 the US National Institute of Occupational Safety and Health evaluated 2,983 fragrance chemicals for health effects. They identified 884 of them as toxic substances. The US EPA found that 100% of perfumes contain toluene, a toxic volatile organic compound (VOC) that can have developmental effects.[37] Toluene is one of the chemicals found in many nail polishes that have caused health problems. Many nail polish manufacturers have removed this chemical from their formulas.*
>
> *Besides toluene, some of the other chemicals used to make fragrances are phthalates, synthetic musks, formaldehyde, and several neurotoxins. One of the reasons the FDA doesn't require that the chemicals that comprise fragrances be individually listed is because a single fragrance can be made up of up to 100 chemicals...they'd*

*need pretty large labels to list them all. So when you buy a fragranced product, there's no way to know what chemicals you've actually purchased and are putting on your body.*

*These chemicals not only cause allergic and irritant reactions in the skin, but they can also be eye irritant, cause or trigger asthma attacks, and damage the immune system.*

*Believe it or not, products marketed as 'unscented' likely contain synthetic chemicals to make them seem like they have no fragrance. The truth is that most ingredients in products have their own scents, and they aren't always pleasant ones.  So manufacturers will use certain chemicals to mask those odors and make give the product a neutral 'un'-scent.*

*The only way to be sure there are no synthetic chemical fragrance ingredients in your products is to either purchase 100% all natural products, or products that say '100% fragrance free', or 'no added fragrance'.*

*What about natural fragrances?*

*Fragrances that are obtained from botanicals such as plant oils, essential oils, extracts, herbs, etc. are generally more tolerated than their synthetic counterparts.  Sure people may have a sensitivity or allergy to a natural ingredient, but it's less likely than with chemical ingredients.  Natural ingredients are often listed individually on labels; so you'll see them there and know if you're allergic or sensitive to it before you purchase it.*

*A natural ingredient will be listed by its botanical name. For example, lavender essential oil is listed as lavandula angustifolia and aloe might be listed as aloe barbadensis.  Be careful though...if you see a natural ingredient listed without the botanical name, or with the word 'fragrance' after it (examples would be 'lavender' or 'lavender fragrance'), you can assume it's not the real natural ingredient, it's a synthetic version of it."*

**Some thoughts regarding preservatives:**

The whole purpose of adding preservatives (any preservatives, regardless of their safety) is to inhibit oxidation and prevent chemical changes that happen to a product due to exposure to air, moisture, contamination from use, or just time itself; which then causes the product to become desirable to microorganisms. Preservatives are necessary in skincare products—even natural, handcrafted ones. All ingredients have the ability to spoil, rot, breed bacteria or other microbes, etc. When a product contains water, as the majority of them do, the chance for contamination and microbial growth grows exponentially. Furthermore, when a product is manufactured in a large batch which will then be stored in a warehouse or stockroom for months to years before ever being opened, preservatives must be added to extend the shelf life.

Not all preservatives are bad—many natural substances like vodka, borax, and essential oils have their own naturally occurring antimicrobial and self-preserving properties. These are the types of preservatives I'm able to use in my own handcrafted products because I produce in tiny batches and can always refrigerate any extra until it's ready for use.

However, that's not the case for mass manufacturers. The chemical preservatives are much stronger and much cheaper to use in mass production, which is why they can make products that have expiration dates 3 years from the batch date. The problem? Many people mistakenly believe that these expiration dates mean that the product is good for 3 years after it's been opened. That isn't the case. Once a product is opened and is exposed to oxygen, moisture, and microbes, it's been contaminated and will begin to spoil quickly regardless of the preservatives it contains. The majority of the chemical preservatives that are used in many commercial products have also been linked to a number of health concerns from skin irritation and allergies all the way to neurotoxicity, endocrine disruption, and even cancer.

While the safety of many skincare ingredients has been questioned, the most controversial ingredients by far are parabens.

## What's the Big Deal About Parabens?[38]

The following is a post I wrote on Holistically Haute™ sharing information I learned about parabens from my aesthetics education and my own research on the subject.

> *"Parabens are antibacterial and anti-fungal, and are supposed to be the least sensitizing preservatives for leave-on topical application. They're also some of the least expensive preservative ingredients that can be used in cosmetic formulations. They stabilize and extend the shelf lives of the products in which they're used. There are many parabens, but the most commonly used ones are methylparaben, ethylparaben, p-propylparaben, isobutylparaben, n-butylparaben and benzylparaben*

> *Why are they bad?*

> *Parabens, have become a topic (and often debate) of great controversy in recent years because of a study conducted by British oncology expert Philippa Darbre. The results were published in 2004. This study[39] found evidence of completely intact parabens in several samples of breast cancer tumor tissues. The results heavily suggested that the parabens were absorbed by the skin, accumulated in the body over time, and produced an overabundance of estrogenic activity which led to breast cancer. There were several limitations of this study, including its small size; but the results were solid enough to warrant extensive further research on the topic.*

> *Since the 2004 study, there have been several others; some suggesting that negatively affect the functions of certain hormones and organs such as androgen and the thyroid..."[40] Dr. Darbre and her colleagues released results from another study in 2008[41] that stated that "the presence of intact paraben esters in human body tissues has now been confirmed by independent measurements in human urine; and the ability of parabens to penetrate human skin intact without breakdown by esterases and to be absorbed systemically has been demonstrated through studies not only in vitro but also in vivo using healthy human*

subjects." Parabens have also been (and continue to be) studied for their effects on the male reproductive system, and other health issues.

On the flip side, there have been a huge number of studies claiming that the use of parabens in small concentrations in cosmetics are safe, because they don't produce a high enough level of estrogenic activity to be harmful, and that they are 'metabolized rapidly by the body and therefore cannot exhibit any adverse effects,'[42] which is contrary to Darbre's research.

So what is the actual risk?

I suppose that is something that you will have to decide for yourself. Whether or not parabens actually cause cancer is the topic of several ongoing studies, and probably won't be confirmed or refuted anytime soon.

All of this research has caused many cosmetic companies to take parabens out of their products and replace them with somewhat safer alternatives, such as ethylhexylglycerin, sorbic acid, potassium sorbate, sodium benzoate, and phenoxyethanol.

Many companies have removed chemical preservatives altogether, instead opting to use blends of highly concentrated plant extracts and essential oils that have naturally occurring antibacterial and antifungal properties; as well as antioxidants that prevent the breakdown and oxidation of a product's ingredients. Colloidal silver is also a good option since it has antimicrobial and germicidal properties.

But many cosmetic manufacturers have elected to keep the parabens in their products. The exact reasons, I don't know for sure. I suspect that a lot of it has to do with keeping manufacturing costs down, and assuming that most of the general public isn't aware of the potential risks posed by parabens.

The fact that many of the companies that still use parabens don't disclose their full ingredient lists on their websites suggests to me that they are fully aware of the potential risks, and that they realize that *more people are also becoming aware; so they don't want people to know that they still use them.*

*If these companies were really so sure that they were safe, then why wouldn't they fully disclose that they use them? I'm sorry, but that is just shady to me. Consumers have the right to know what is inside their products, and they should be able to have a choice on whether or not they want to purchase paraben-containing products.*

*It all comes down to this: **All types of cancer are on the rise.** More people today get some type of cancer than ever before. I don't know a single person who hasn't been affected by cancer in some way. Many of the causes of cancer are things we have little to no control over, such as genetic predisposition and environmental toxins and pollution, but there are some risks we can reduce or eliminate.*

*I've seen too many people's lives taken from them or changed forever because of cancer. To me, avoiding parabens and other ingredients that have any level of cancer risk at all is a no-brainer. **If I can do something that cuts my risk of getting cancer even a little bit, then why wouldn't I do that?** That doesn't just include avoiding parabens...it involves making healthy choices in all areas of nutrition and lifestyle."*

In addition to parabens, there are several other ingredients that are huge red flags for toxicity. I'd seen several lists of with different chemical ingredients to avoid such as "The Toxic 12" and "The Dirty 30." I thought I'd be a smarty and compile my own top 30 ingredients to avoid (though the list goes on way past 30):

1. **Parabens**
2. **Petroleum and other petrochemicals**
3. **Synthetic fragrances**
4. **Sulfates** (sodium and ammonium laureth/lauryl sulfates)
5. **Phthalates** AKA dibutyl phthalate (DBP), 2-ethylhexyl phthalate (DEHP) diethyl phthalate (DEP), butyl benzyl phthalate
6. **Lead** (lead acetate)
7. **Mercury** (thimerosol or Merthiolate®)

8. **Hydroquinone**
9. **Triclosan**
10. **Toluene** AKA toluol, methylbenzene
11. **Xylene** AKA xylol or dimethylbenzene
12. **BHA and BHT** (Butylated hydroxyanisole and butylated hydroxytoluene, respectively)
13. **Propylene Glycol**
14. **Dyes such as coal tar dyes, p-phenylenediamine (PPD), "Colour Index" or "CI" colors**
15. **DEA, MEA, TEA** (not tea the drink)
16. **Formaldehyde and formaldehyde-releasing preservatives** (DMDM hydantoin, diazolidinyl urea, imidazolidinyl urea, methenamine, and quarternium-15)
17. **PEG (polyethylene glycol) compounds**
18. **Siloxanes and most other silicones**
19. **Nano- and micronized particles**
20. **Talc**
21. **Chemical sunscreens** such as oxybenzone
22. **Retinoic acid** (Retin-A®)
23. **Isotretinoin** (Accutane®)
24. **Corticosteroids**
25. **Glycolic acid**
26. **Salicylic acid**
27. **Benzoyl peroxide**
28. **Talc/talcum powder**
29. **Benzene**
30. **Aluminum powder**
31. **Resorcinol**

## Why should I care about topical skincare ingredients?

It's important because what a lot of people don't realize is that even though the skin is a strong barrier on its best day, we still absorb up to 60% of what we put on topically. So people think that just because they putting it on their skin—they're not ingesting it—that it's not going into the body. That's not true. Many of us have compromised skin anyway so it's likely that we might be absorbing more than that 60%; therefore a large amount of the chemicals that are in the skincare will enter the body. Once inside, they can accumulate over time and produce a toxic reaction.

Using harsh and toxic ingredients on the skin, especially for prolonged periods of time, can lead to permanent damage topically and internally. Certain acids, like glycolic and salicylic may cause serious chemical burns to the skin. Certain preservatives and other agents release formaldehyde, which is a known carcinogen. Synthetic fragrances and detergents can cause irritation, inflammation, and have other reactions in the body so it's really important to use skincare ingredients that are appropriate for your skin type, and are safe and gentle.

**Enough of that serious talk! Let's talk about something more fun—your skincare regimen.**

I know skincare products can be pricey, and with all of the marketing and hype out there it is hard to know if you're actually getting a quality product that will work. So here are some ways you can save money on your regimen.

What I'm about to tell you is going to sound a bit counterintuitive:

Buy higher quality products that have higher quality ingredients in them. I know, I know—higher quality ingredients and products are more expensive! However, since the ingredients are both more potent and more bioavailable, these products are going to be much more effective. Remember this: *the most expensive product is the one that does not work—or worse—the one that causes a serious irritant or allergic reaction.* Always choose quality over quantity.

I think it's also really smart to have a set skincare budget in mind, and also have an idea of how involved you want to get with it. In my past life, I was at the point where I was using seven or eight products on my face twice a day and it got really expensive. I thought I really needed this, this, and this and of course the advertisements said that the products were all "formulated to work together" so before I knew it, I needed a second job just to pay for my monthly skincare! You have to be smart, and you have to not be swayed by marketing.

Still, many people enjoy using a variety of products and benefit from using certain formulations—for example, eye creams are formulated with smaller molecules that are designed to penetrate the skin around the eyes that has fewer and smaller pores than the rest of the face. I realize that a lot of people think eye cream is a big scam, and that it's not a necessary or effective product. I have to tell you though, I'm a believer in eye cream. I've been using eye cream since I was 22 years old and I really do think that's the reason I don't have any lines around my eyes at 36.

Another example is serum. Serums are formulated with very high concentrations of active ingredients for targeted concerns—usually for anti-aging, but there are also serums specifically developed with acne-fighting ingredients.

For people with specific goals that are OK with adding one or two additional products to their regimen, I typically recommend a cleanser, toner, serum, eye cream, day cream containing a natural sunscreen (or a tinted moisturizer with a natural sunscreen), and a moisturizer for nighttime that does not contain sun protection. That's what I use personally.

But if you're really on a tight budget or you don't have (or want to spend) the time with all of those products, you can look for products that multitask like a cleansing oil or lotion cleanser and a tinted moisturizer with sunscreen. I know plenty of people who use an oil like jojoba with some essential oils for both cleansing and moisturizing and they do just fine.

### Where should I buy my skincare products?

I highly recommend that people experiment and make products themselves, but if you're not ready to dive into that yet, then I recommend a specialty health-minded store like Whole Foods Market or somewhere similar. These stores often offer a fairly good selection of skincare products containing safer, more natural ingredients. You could also try local craft fairs and farmers market, as they often have local artisans and vendors of natural, handcrafted products.

This isn't going to be a popular statement, but I don't really like many of the brands at department stores or even the specialty cosmetics stores. These stores are chock full of mass marketed, mass produced, chemical-laden products and offer very few, if any, safe and natural alternatives.

Many people assume that products from dermatologists' offices and medical spas are automatically safe and are more effective. While they do contain higher quantities of pharmaceutical grade, active ingredients, many of these "medical" products tend to be quite harsh. If it's affordable, I would suggest going to a holistically-minded spa and asking for products that are free of the nasty ingredients—ask specifically for the terms "paraben-free, sulfate-free, free of synthetic fragrances," etc. Fortunately, there are a lot of really nice spa quality skincare brands that are free of the harmful chemicals these days. The trends seem to be shifting away from the harsher chemicals and into more holistic and organic ingredients. Again you just have to do your homework. It depends on your budget too—obviously the spa products are going to be more expensive than the stuff at Whole Foods.

How I personally save money on my skincare products is that I make them myself. I experimented in my kitchen for quite some time and I've come up with my own formulations that work better on my skin than anything I've ever used before. I buy all the raw materials in bulk from online suppliers, and the cost is a sliver of what I used to pay. So if you are creative, if you like to cook and are willing to experiment, that's the best way to save money on your products.

**How effective are homemade skincare products and how easy are they to make?**

They are as easy to make as cooking, really, once you get the right recipe. I really enjoy it and it really doesn't take that long—only a few minutes once you know what recipe you want to use. It did take me a little while to come up with my basic recipes, but I'm glad I took the time because they are very effective! I've been using my own products exclusively for the last 2 years and not only is my bank account happy with me but my skin is too because it looks better than it ever has.

I think these products are more effective because the ingredients are undiluted and minimally (if at all) processed. As we discussed before, when you buy a mass-marketed product, you are mostly getting water then a mass of chemicals to prevent bacterial growth; very little actual active ingredients. So the products that I make using all natural ingredients are very rich with nutrients, contain very little water, and I only produce how much I need at a time so there is really no need for preservatives.

## Special Bonus Just for You!

Because I really want you to try to make your own products yourself, I've put together some of my favorite cleansing oil recipes and list of preferred online suppliers that you can download at www.holisticallyhaute.com/love-your-skin-bonus-recipes.html FREE as my gift to you. You will love these, regardless of your skin type.

**Why would I use an oil based product if my skin is already oily?**

The idea that people with oily or broken out skin can't use oils to cleanse and moisturize the skin is one of the biggest myths out there. The fact is that many oils, like the ones we discussed above that mimic human sebum, don't clog the pores and don't create a greasy residue on the skin. These oils dissolve dirt, debris, and makeup to leave the skin clean, hydrated, and nourished while leaving its protective barrier intact. This helps to actually regulate the skin's production of sebum, because the skin isn't constantly in reactive mode from being dehydrated by harsh detergents. Jojoba, argan, rosehip seed, sweet almond, and kukui nut oil are great examples of these oils.

This concept applies to essential oils as well. The term "essential oil" is actually a misnomer because most of them are not oily or greasy at all.

**5 of my favorite essential oils to use in skincare products and their therapeutic properties[43]:**

- **Melaleuca (tea tree oil):** While the aroma of this oil might be an acquired taste, it's excellent for acne and other skin infections due to its antibacterial, antifungal, antiviral, and anti-inflammatory properties. It also helps to stimulate the immune system and regenerate damaged tissue.
- **Lavender:** This is my favorite aroma and my favorite essential oil because it's so universal. It's anti-inflammatory, analgesic, regenerative, and sedative which makes it very good for soothing irritated, inflamed conditions like rosacea, psoriasis, and eczema. It also is antimicrobial which makes it good to add to acne blends.
- **Frankincense:** This ancient oil has anti-infectious, anti-inflammatory, antiseptic, immune system stimulating, and sedative effects as well. It benefits all skin conditions and also works synergistically with other oils in blends.
- **Geranium:** This is a great one to add to any blend containing melaleuca, because it masks its scent well. Geranium is also antibacterial and sedative, but is also astringent and tonic which is great for acne or seborrhea.
- **Roman chamomile:** This oil is best known for its calming and relaxing properties in addition to being anti-inflammatory and anti-infectious. It's excellent for dermatitis, eczema, or rashes.

### Your internal skincare regimen: This is completely optional, but extremely beneficial!

You may have heard the term "nutriceutical" in terms of supplements. "Nutriceutical" is a fancy word for "supplement that benefits the skin." That's where the idea of treating the skin from the inside out came from. These are internal vitamins, minerals, antioxidants, and proteins that you take in the form of a capsule, powder, or liquid that ideally (if sourced from high-quality, whole foods and are formulated properly) deliver high concentrations of targeted nutrients to the skin cells as they are forming.

The most popular ones I've come across are the proteins collagen and hyaluronic acid, as well as antioxidants like Pycnogenol ®, resveratrol, and alpha lipoic acid. I'm going to discuss the proteins in more detail because they are harder to get from whole food sources in high quantities since the supplements are sourced from animal parts that we don't typically like to eat. The antioxidants are much easier to obtain through a diet rich in fresh, raw fruits and vegetables.

Collagen is one of the most important proteins found in the body. It's very strong and pliable, and supports our bones, joints, and connective tissues including the skin. Collagen makes up about 70% of the dermis (deeper layer of the skin), and is produced by cells called fibroblasts. As we age, these cells produce less and less collagen and elastin, another important protein fiber that supports the skin. The collagen within the dermis begins to deplete causing the dermis to thin out as part of the skin's aging process. Poor lifestyle choices like smoking, excessive UV exposure, toxic build-up, poor diet, dehydration, and stress actually speed up the degradation of collagen, causing premature aging in the skin, as well as in the body, which leads to joint pain and brittle hair and nails. Conversely, making healthy diet and lifestyle choices can help preserve collagen and encourage the body to keep producing this essential protein fiber. While the only direct whole food sources of collagen are muscles, bones, and tendons of cows, as well as the bones of certain fish, diets high in fruits and vegetables that contain Vitamin C will help the body synthesize more collagen on its own. This doesn't happen overnight, of course, which is why a high-quality collagen supplement might be desirable.

Hyaluronic acid (HA) is another protein abundant in our skin and bodies at birth, but degrades as we age. It's unique because of its extreme humectant properties, meaning its ability to draw and retain water. It's quite possibly the most powerful humectant due to its capacity to hold 1,000 times its own molecular weight in water. It also has antioxidant benefits. This is what makes it such a hot commodity in skincare formulations: not only does it provide extreme hydration to the skin, it also pushes other active ingredients deeper into the skin while allowing it to breathe at the same time (unlike certain emollients and heavy occlusives). HA is also quite a popular internal supplement these days and is often marketed as a nutriceutical as well as for joint health with similar indications as glucosamine chondroitin/sulfate supplements. There are some vegetable sources of hyaluronic acid (also known as sodium hyaluronate or hyaluronon), such as dark leafy greens, beets, beans, nuts, seeds, starchy vegetables, and certain fruits that are high in magnesium and zinc, but you'd have to eat large quantities of these foods to get a concentration of HA high enough to affect a dramatic improvement in the skin or joints.

Again, while supplements are never meant to be substitutions for a healthy, well-balanced, whole food-based diet, they can help maximize the benefits of certain nutrients and proteins.

As with topical skincare products, you have to do your homework with nutriceuticals, as well as any internal supplement or multivitamin. Angel dusting occurs in the supplement industry, and there are a lot of low-quality synthetics in many of the lower-priced, nationally advertised brands. I really do believe that you get what you pay for and when a product is heavily advertised, you can assume that's where the majority of that company's money is going and not so much into sourcing the highest quality ingredients. Don't be afraid to go to your local health food store or farmers' markets to see what they have to offer. You might find something interesting—like a seaweed supplement that might be really good for the skin. These places often have unique topical products as well. Keep in mind that in general, nutriceuticals and supplements are only effective if they come from a very high-quality source.

**Let's talk hygiene.**

So many people overwash and overscrub their skin! Remember, you simply want to wash away any dirt, makeup, or accumulated excess oil and debris on the surface—you're not scrubbing grout in your bathroom tile.

I always recommend that you wash your face before bed, especially if you wear makeup. It's never a good idea to sleep with makeup. Even if it is one of the newer mineral formulations that claims to be so pure you can sleep with it. Don't do it. It hardly takes any time at all to wash your face at night, especially if you use a cleansing oil. Most makeup is oil- or wax-based, as is debris that collects on the surface and in the pores. Like attracts like, and the natural plant oils will attract and dissolve the dirt and makeup so you can easily (and gently) wipe it clean, quickly.

It's nice to wash your face in the morning just to help you wake up and freshen up, but face it—your skin isn't really getting all that filthy while you are sleeping. It might get oily, so if you have oilier skin it's nice to use a very gentle cleanser, lotion cleanser, or cleansing oil, but not a harsh, foaming cleanser.

You know that "squeaky clean feeling?" That's actually not a good thing—it means that you've stripped away your skin's natural moisturizing factor with ingredients (usually surfactants and detergents) that are too harsh. This doesn't make your skin cleaner, and it's really troublesome for people with oilier skin because by over-stripping the skin's natural protective oils, the skin goes into panic mode and overcompensates by producing more oil. Some people with drier skin actually get irritated by washing too much.

While good skin hygiene certainly includes washing your face, there are several other aspects of hygiene that are just as important but often left out:

- **Clean makeup brushes often.** This is really important and a lot of people don't do it nearly enough. Brushes contaminated with old, oily, caked-on, dead skin cells and residues of sebum and makeup are playgrounds for bacteria, viruses, and fungi. I suggest washing them in warm water with a gentle cleanser and letting them air dry once a week.
- **Changing pillow cases often is crucial, especially if you have acne.** Once a week is fine for people without an inflammatory skin condition, but if you do have acne or another type of lesion or infection, change your pillow cases several times a week.
- **Keep your hands off of your face!** So many people touch their faces several times throughout the day without even realizing it. Doing this puts all that dirt and nastiness from the hands onto already compromised skin (if you have a condition).
- **Resist the urge to pick.** I know, I know...those big, ripe, white pustules are just begging to be popped. And those blackheads seem to stare back at you in the mirror like little, taunting

eyeballs—they need to be stopped! It's so tempting to pick or attempt to extract blackheads, whiteheads, dry patches, and scabs, but the more you pick, the more you risk spreading infection and causing permanent scarring and broken capillaries. It's a much better—and safer—idea to get a deep cleaning facial at a spa and have extractions done professionally to minimize negative effects. At home, you can try using an absorbing clay-based mask once a week, which will help pull the impurities out of the skin.

- **Don't over-scrub the skin, especially if you have acne, eczema, psoriasis, or rosacea.** It's only going to make the condition worse. I know it's hard to resist scrubbing at the scaly lesions that come with eczema and psoriasis, but that's not the way to get rid of them. All scrubbing will do is make them more inflamed, which will slow down the healing process.
- **Change and launder washcloths and towels after every use** because they can collect molds and bacteria, which you don't want to be rubbing on your skin.

# Chapter 10: Self Image and Healing on the Inside

Developing a strong sense of self-worth, self-esteem, self-image, and self-love is challenging enough for women in a society that thrusts images of flawless perfection in our faces at every turn. As adults, we can intellectually understand that most of these images are manipulated in some way—but even though we know this in our heads, we don't always know it in our hearts. For some reason, we still feel that our own real life images should match the false ones presented as today's "ideal" woman. Somehow, the idea that beauty is in the eye of the beholder becomes skewed when the majority of what's beheld is not reality. This makes it very challenging to be the beholder, who though she is likely very beautiful in many ways, only sees her flaws (even when no one else does) because she doesn't have the smooth, well-lit, perfectly coifed and made up reflection of the models and actresses she sees on TV and in movies .

Many women lack self-love and a positive self-image—they don't need to have a visible skin condition to have this outlook since society does such a fine job of it on its own. However, when you have a skin condition that elicits a reaction from other people, it validates the feelings of low self-image. While we are our own worst critics, when others' glances and comments send the message, "Yes! You do have horrible skin! I don't want to get too close to you because I don't want to catch anything!" it adds a challenge to each day that begins as soon as you wake up and glance in the mirror.

I started getting acne when I was about 10 years old. Back then, it wasn't all that visible to others, but it was noticeable at times. When I got my first pimple, I was actually excited because it came shortly after "the talk" about puberty at school—you know, when the girls are shown a cheesy film and sent home with maxi pads while the boys talked about who knows what with the male gym teacher. That talk meant I was finally growing up and would not be a "kid" much longer. Soon would come the days of bras and periods (if I only knew at the time how super fun those would be!), and then of course dating and other cool teenage girl stuff that I read about in *YM* magazine and my *Sweet Valley High* and *Babysitters Club books.* That pimple was proof to me that I was on my way. That feeling lasted about a week. That's when more pimples and blackheads began to appear and I started realizing that maybe growing up wasn't all it was cracked up to be.

I became really self-conscious because I didn't notice my friends' skin breaking out. At that time it wasn't noticeable enough that people made fun of me, but in my own head, I started to feel that people were staring at me. It affected me even at that age. As I got older and started going through puberty, the acne became quite severe. My skin ran the full gamut—sometimes I'd have lots of large blackheads, which then turned into raised, red bumps (papules) or larger, inflamed whiteheads (pustules), and even larger and quite painful cysts, which lie underneath the surface of the skin and don't come to the surface or "pop" when you squeeze them. I squeezed them anyway, and always ended up breaking the skin and getting scabs, and later, scars, which of course made it all worse.

I became the quintessential "pizza face" girl. It was awful. People were mean. In junior high school, I was at band practice (I played the clarinet) and I remember feeling eyes on me coming from my left. I looked at the girl sitting there and she was staring at my face with a look of confusion and disgust. "What?" I asked. "Nothing..." she said. After a pause she asked, "Actually...what's wrong with your face?" I was mortified, especially since other people heard the conversation. That's when things really started to go downhill. I always felt like I had to hide, like there was something wrong with me. One of my first boyfriends said to me, "I love you—I even love your zits." Um, thank you?

I felt like a freak and was called names like "zit face" and "leper." I overheard teachers, parents, even doctors, say stuff like, "Oh she's such a pretty girl, it's a shame she has that all over her face," or "she'd be so much prettier if it wasn't for those pimples." Adults who make these types of comments about or to adolescents often claim to mean well, but they obviously don't know how hurtful it actually is to be a kid or young woman who's already having a hard time trying to figure out who she is; or rather, who she is supposed to be.

Even on "good skin days," I always felt like I had to cover it up, or that people were staring or judging me. I became too nervous to make eye contact for fear that the person would turn away and wonder, "oh my God was she just looking at me?" I have a confession. I wanted to date the boys in my school—there were several I had crushes on—but I was so afraid they thought I was grotesque I rarely attempted to talk to any of them. I still really wanted to date though, and I had friends in other schools, so almost all of my high school relationships began as phone calls with boys from other schools that turned into blind dates, which eventually became relationships. I felt safe talking to these guys on the phone—like I could be myself and I felt they liked me enough after getting to know me on the phone that when we met in person, they wouldn't care about my skin (which, of course I covered with layers of concealer, foundation, and powder).

Throughout this painful time, I always had hope that it would be over in a few short years. When my acne persisted into adulthood, I was pissed off! I was always told, "Oh it's going to go away, it will get better, don't worry; it's just a phase, you'll grow out of it." Well, I didn't and I was so frustrated! It's even worse as an adult because then people think, "What's wrong with her that she still has acne?"

Though my poor self-image issues developed in my teen years, they progressed into more serious issues in college and into young adulthood. This became very apparent in my relationships—particularly with men. I always wondered, "Is this guy going to be attracted to me for me? He can't possibly be attracted to my face because I'm so disgusting. He must only want me for my body, or maybe I only deserve a certain type of man because I have this on my face. Maybe I'm not worth a man who has perfect skin. Could a man really love me despite having this skin?" I made a lot of very poor choices because of these feelings and thoughts. I surrounded myself with people who didn't support me or help me move forward in a positive direction.

These thought processes were very damaging. I questioned people's motives, and even when I'd find a good person, even my now husband, I doubted them. These issues were so deeply seated in my thought process that they even got in the way of my ability to form good friendships and positive relationships with co-workers. When you don't have a good or realistic view of yourself, your own reality becomes askew and your view of others is affected. It hinders your ability to relate and communicate.

**Does it matter what people think?**

Sure, it matters when you are a teenager trying to fit into the popular clique and date the hot varsity athlete. But many adults are still trying to fit in too—at work, with friends, even within their own families. As much as we don't want to admit that we care what people think, we do. A lot of people say "I don't care what they think, I don't care what you think, I'm fine the way I am." That sounds good, but when you've convinced yourself that everyone is staring at you, gossiping about you, or judging you based on your appearance, it matters.

Even if you're one of the lucky ones who has outgrown the skin condition, it might still be affecting you emotionally. Confidence is a huge issue for adults with active and even resolved skin conditions. Maybe you worry that you'll be passed over for a job promotion because you're too self-conscious to give a good presentation at work, for example. Some feel too self-conscious about their appearance to look someone else in the eye, or trust that they are genuine. While it "shouldn't" matter what others think, it really does matter to people who are experiencing these thoughts and emotions. It's easy for people on the outside to say, "Oh what do you care what people say or think?" But when you're the person who's actually dealing with these insecurities, it matters very much. Especially when it's coming from people you love who are supposed to love you; they're the ones whose approval is most needed.

**Self-image and skin problems**

Skin problems can affect people very deeply in several ways. I have worked with many women whose skin conditions have dampened their ability to truly live joyful and fulfilled lives. Below are the stories of women I've worked with, whose skin conditions affected their lives. Names have been changed for privacy.

*Karen is a young woman who developed acne as an adult but never had it as a teenager. She'd been to doctors, and had tests done, but none of them found anything wrong with her. One doctor prescribed her birth control pills to help reduce breakouts by regulating her hormones, but all this did was mess with her moods and give her melasma. She went off the pills, but the acne and melasma persisted. At some points, her breakouts were so bad that she didn't want to leave her house. She missed a lot of work because of this and was afraid of losing her job. She felt completely lost and confused about why this was happening to her, and she was afraid that her new husband would no longer be attracted to her. She was ridden with anxiety and couldn't sleep. She spent a fortune on doctors, medications, and products and just wanted to look and feel like herself again. Karen completed a 6-month holistic skincare coaching program with me. After 1 month, she began sleeping again. After 2 months, her acne was clear and she was no longer missing work. By the end of her program, the melasma improved dramatically and she felt like she had reclaimed her old self.*

*Mary is a holistic nurse in her early fifties. She is in the beginning stages of menopause and during a hot flash, noticed that her skin became extremely red and blotchy on her nose, cheeks, chin, and chest. At first, she thought it was because of the hot flash, but became concerned when the redness did not fade for hours after the hot flash subsided. She began to experience these flare ups more frequently, sometimes accompanied by hot flashes, and realized she had developed rosacea. Even when she didn't have the redness, she had visible broken capillaries on her nose and cheeks all the time. The flare ups were unpredictable, and she began to feel self-conscious when working with patients, because holistic health practitioners are supposed to be healthy. She went through her diet to try to identify triggers and did extensive research on different causes of rosacea, but was overwhelmed with all the information. She didn't want to go on hormones* or steroids for the rosacea (or menopause) but the fear of flare ups caused her to stop pursuing new clients for her holistic nursing practice because she felt like a fraud. People around her noticed her skin condition, and she felt judged. Though Mary already had extensive knowledge of diet and lifestyle choices, she felt very alone and overwhelmed about where to start to heal her condition. After 3 months of what I like to refer to as, "structured trial and error," in addition to some in-depth health, lifestyle, and spiritual coaching, Mary and I were able to identify foods and other triggers that not only triggered the rosacea flare ups, but also the hot flashes. She has resumed growing her holistic nursing practice and has also lost weight during the process.

*Kelly is a college professor and mother of a teenage girl. She says her skin has been "confused" since her teenage years with very large pores and blackheads on her nose and chin, oily eyelids, and extremely dry and scaly in the corners of her mouth and eyes as well as on her scalp (dandruff). She also would get patches of eczema on her hands periodically. She was always very self-conscious of her dandruff while a student and was called "Flakes" by the mean girls at her school. The scaly areas around her eyes and mouth were so easily irritated that they would crack, ooze, and bleed at the slightest facial expression. She was afraid to laugh or frown, so she avoided people and conversations; she went through high school and college with no friends. She'd gotten used to her avoidance routine, but when her teenage daughter began to develop similar symptoms, she knew she didn't want her daughter to grow up feeling as isolated as she did, so she sought my help. Early on, we were able to identify several areas of her diet and lifestyle that were possible contributors to her skin's "confused" state. By making small adjustments, we were able to dramatically improve the dandruff and scaling around her face and mouth within 3 months. At the end of our 6 months together, she felt that she looked 10 years younger and she began to love smiling at herself in the mirror. More importantly, she helped her daughter make the same adjustments, and her daughter's symptoms disappeared after 1 month and haven't come back.*

**Healing skin conditions is the holistic way to heal the emotional issues caused by them.**

One of the things I noticed after working with so many women with skin concerns is that their self-image issues were caused by their skin condition, and rarely by something else as might be the case with emotional eating or an eating disorder. Those problems are fairly mainstream and have a variety of different treatment protocols available ranging from holistic to medical.

This isn't really the case with skin conditions, because the notion that what you eat and how you live can affect the skin isn't yet fully accepted by mainstream medicine or even conventional aesthetics. While emotions of guilt and self-sabotage might exist in an overweight person, most people with skin conditions aren't aware that something in their diet or lifestyle may have caused their condition. Therefore, there aren't really feelings of guilt or questions of whether or not they somehow caused their condition because most people believe it's just a fact of life, or that it's due to family history. When you heal the skin physically, you can start to heal emotionally too. You look in the mirror and see someone with beautiful skin looking back at you.

I like to use the comparison of systemic inflammation to describe it. Inflammation in the body causes several health concerns: autoimmune diseases, cardiovascular diseases, respiratory diseases, etc. However, these aren't issues that you can necessarily see in a mirror, so you usually think nothing of them. While inflammation certainly might affect your quality of life, without constant, visible reminders, it's not something that necessarily keeps you up at night. You also don't really have to wonder if people are whispering "Wow check out that girl's high blood pressure! Something must be wrong with her."

However, you see a skin condition every time you look in a mirror or pass a window. It's also everybody's first impression of you. It's not something you think you have control over and sometimes, in fact, you might not have control over it. You feel almost like you are under attack or being punished. You wonder why this is happening to you when so many other people don't have these issues.

It took me a really long time to understand that my own self-image issues were actually a result of my skin issues. I had gone to a variety of therapists who suggested that I was depressed or had social anxiety, but none of them could explain why.

Even back then, I didn't understand how a mental health issue could just appear from nowhere. I knew it was a response to something; I just couldn't put my finger on what. It wasn't until years later, when I began to see improvements in my skin after changing my diet, lifestyle, and skincare regimen that I realized that I was actually fine. By eliminating the cause (the bad skin), I immediately began to see myself differently every day. It took a while, because it was weird to only spend 10 minutes on my makeup rather than 45. I was so used to spending time in the mirror squeezing pimples and blackheads that not seeing them after a while became a bit alarming.

It took quite a while for me to be able to accept compliments from people. Even recently, if I get complimented on a nice photograph, I still am quick to give credit to the photographer or to the lighting, or say that I was wearing colors that flattered me so that's why the picture came out so well. It wasn't until I saw my last batch of headshots and realized that they didn't need any retouching at all that I realized that it was because of me— not the camera, not the lights—just me. It was a revelation! I couldn't stop staring at my photos and smiling—I even apologized to the friend I was with at the studio because I was pretty vocal about how much I loved the pictures. There may have even been singing involved.

**Learning to truly love yourself is an important step in changing your skin... and your life.**

When you begin to prioritize yourself and recognize that you deserve love and care just as much as everyone else does, that you don't have to look to others to receive that love and care, it makes all the difference. Any love or validation you seek from others will never fill the void—the only way to do that is to first find it within yourself.

Like anything worthwhile in life, it may not come easy to find love and validation when you are harder on yourself than anyone else. It will likely require you to emerge from the cocoon of safety you've been hiding in for so long. The thought of facing the judgment you've been hiding from is terrifying.

**Ask yourself these questions:**

1. Am I happy living my life like this?

2. What would my life be like if these thoughts and fears were no longer there?

3. What am I missing out on because of my lack of self-confidence, longing to hide, or low self-image?

4. Was I given this life to live in fear and misery?

Remember—continuing on the same path will never lead you to a new destination. You have to take a different path—sometimes you have to carve out your own path. And that's really OK, because a path that you've created yourself will always lead you to where you're meant to go. I truly believe that.

**It's time to come out of hibernation and emerge. Do this now:**

Go outside. It doesn't matter if it's day or night, warm or cold, raining or clear. Go outside and stretch your arms up to the heavens. Lengthen your spine, open your heart, root your feet and imagine the light from the sun or the moon washing over you. Breathe in deeply and breathe out loudly. Say outloud:

"I'm awake now. I'm here and from this moment I'm going to LIVE my life." Saying it to yourself in your head is OK at first, but the louder you say this, the more real your intention will be. It doesn't matter if the neighbors can hear you. Even if they do, they'll probably respond, "You go, girl!" The more you do this, the more you'll believe it to be true. This is your first step to taking control of your own life, your own happiness, and your own destiny.

You are now awake and can begin to be aware.

While you're healing from any condition, whether it's physical, emotional, or even spiritual (or all three—they're interconnected) it's important to master the skill of self-awareness. One of the first ways to increase self-awareness is to give yourself permission to feel your feelings and experience your emotions without labeling or censoring them.

What does this mean? Imagine you're waiting for a phone call from the human resources representative of a company where you just interviewed for a new job. You know the call will come in the afternoon and you are sitting by the phone chewing a pencil and drumming your fingernails. What are you feeling? Nervous? Anxious? Afraid? A little bit nauseous? Excited?

Do you allow yourself to attach other thoughts, labels, or unrealistic expectations to those emotions? For example: "I'm afraid I won't get the job because I'm not experienced enough" or "I'm excited to get this job because it will change my life for the better." By attaching these specific labels to the emotions, you're potentially setting yourself up for disappointment, which can negatively affect your self-esteem and self-worth. Instead, allow yourself to just sit in the emotion and observe it. If you're feeling anxious, what does that mean? Are there any other words you can use to describe the feeling besides "anxious?" Bring your awareness into your body. Are you clenching anything or are you feeling pain or discomfort anywhere? Does this feeling remind you of a particular memory, image, or even a color? Going through this process of deconstructing your emotion without judging or censoring it is a proactive way to take control of your emotions and the situation at hand. Regardless of whether you get the job or not, you've made huge progress in facing a potentially scary emotion head on and dealing with it constructively.

Another way to hone your self-awareness is to communicate your feelings to someone you trust—someone who won't judge you or even necessarily give you advice—but will offer a safe space for you and listen without interrupting. If that's not possible, journaling is a really powerful tool to explore your emotions and the physical sensations or experiences you might be having.

When I first began to recover from my physical and emotional conditions,

I found my strongest relief through creative expression because I was allowing myself to feel proud of my creations. Creating beautiful things helped me realize that I had beauty inside of me, even if I couldn't yet see it in the mirror—what you create from scratch is a reflection of who you really are. Healing has a great deal to do with making consistently conscious choices–choosing not to be a victim, choosing to put yourself out there, choosing to ask for help, choosing to explore and channel emotions, and choosing to honor your body and your spirit with positive thoughts and acts.

Cultivating self-awareness and choosing to be present in your life and with the people around you improves the way you relate to other people because you radiate a different energy. When you emit more positive energy, you'll attract more positive people into your life. They're going to want to be around you more and you'll feel better about what you have to offer to the world. You're a crucial part of a much greater whole. Realizing your importance and owning your worth affects everyone around you, which then creates a ripple effect. You have the ability to make a difference in many people's lives.

Overcoming self-image issues that stem from skin conditions can be challenging and it takes time. That's OK! Even after a skin condition is physically healed, a lot of emotional stuff may still remain for years to come, whether they're issues from childhood or more recent problems that began in adulthood.

I wasn't fully aware of the preconceived notions that I'd developed as a result of my skin condition until quite recently as I began making some changes in my business and re-evaluated why I was doing certain things. It became very clear to me that I really hadn't quite healed from my own self-image issues because I still questioned if I was "good" enough and still had a constant need to be validated and receive external approval. Once I was aware that I had these needs and tendencies, I worked through them using yoga, meditation, mindfulness, journaling, as well as talking with a very close friend who I trust completely with even my most raw and unreasonable emotions.

Once I realized that self-love and positive self-image are choices, my skin, my weight, my relationships with others, my career, and my entire quality of life improved dramatically. Having bad skin at some point in your life might leave you with physical and emotional scars, but it's not a death sentence and it's not a life sentence; it's something that can be overcome. You have the ability to choose to love yourself; even if you don't fully believe it yet, the more you put it out there, the sooner you will realize it to be true. The more you practice it, the more it becomes real.

I also want to drive home the point that cleaning up your diet not only helps physically heal your skin, it also can change the way your mind processes thoughts. Eating healthier foods does tend to make people happier.

**So now I'm a little bit older and I have my own children.**

I had to find a way to be a woman and mother with self-image and skin issues and have the courage to be a positive role model for my children. I think that if you're a mother of children—boys or girls—it's important for them to see you taking good care of yourself, and presenting yourself confidently, because that's what they are going to emulate.

I intend to help my children avoid growing up with the same skin and self-image issues that I went through—that's actually part of the reason why I went to school for aesthetics. I wanted to learn how to spot signs of acne early on in my children and have the knowledge and tools to nip it in the bud before it became a problem that affected them physically or emotionally. I'll be damned if I let acne or any other skin condition ravage or destroy my children's beautiful skin and beautiful souls. Not gonna happen, not on my watch.

The best way is to start them young on a healthy diet regimen and proper hygiene. I can't stress it enough. This is where my tough love side comes out because I feel so strongly about it. As a parent and a health coach, I've heard all the excuses in the world about how the kids don't want to eat the vegetables and they don't want to drink water they want to drink juice, they want candy—I don't want to hear it. I become really frustrated when I hear the excuses because, parents: these are your children. They didn't ask to be born. You chose to bring them into this world and it's your responsibility to do everything in your power to make sure that they grow up to be healthy, happy, balanced human beings.

I used to be an excuse-making parent as well. For years, my little one wouldn't eat fruits and vegetables. I eventually stopped offering them because it was easier to just feed her something else and avoid the whining. I realized later on that by giving in, I was letting her control the situation, which I knew was wrong since I'm the parent and she's the child. If I let her control situations as a toddler, I knew I'd be completely screwed once she becomes a teenager!

I then made the decision to get rid of the foods I didn't want my kids to have anymore. They didn't like it at first, but guess what? It didn't take that long for them to adjust. Now my stubborn little one eats fruits and vegetables daily and will try anything I put in front of her. It's so important to teach your kids good habits when they're young because the younger they are, the less they'll resist you. The older they are, the longer the bad habits have been present, the harder it's going to be—but fear not, it's still doable.

**Another tough love moment: check that attitude.**

Having a positive attitude can either propel you forward on your journey to healthier skin and a happier life, or it can keep you stuck in your cocoon. It's your choice. We mustn't give into the victim mentality. It's important that we assess the situation and see it for what it is in reality without creating drama or placing blame on your parents, the mean girls, God, or anyone else. Nobody's punishing you and nobody did this to you. There's nothing wrong with you and you're not a freak. If you don't have the knowledge to take care of the condition right now and what you're doing is not working, you need to take responsibility, get on the Internet, go to an aesthetician, go to a holistic practitioner, even go to a doctor if it means getting more information about your condition. Just try something different. Don't be complacent and just go through the motions of life. Remember, there's no reason to be miserable if you're not going to do something to change your situation. You have to make the choice that you don't want to live this way anymore.

# Chapter 11: Your Path Begins – the Future is Bright and Beautiful!

When I first made the commitment to change things in my life, I felt afraid, nervous, doubtful, frustrated, excited, overwhelmed, anxious, confused—you name it, I felt it. Once I realized how much of a commitment and total lifestyle overhaul would be necessary, I wasn't sure I was ready for it, but I knew that whatever "it" was had to be better than how I was feeling.

The most challenging part for me was that I truly felt alone. My family and friends thought my choices to dump my chemical-containing products and radically change my diet were extreme and a bit insane. They couldn't understand why I would voluntarily cut out dairy products if I was never diagnosed with casein allergy or lactose intolerance. The same was true with gluten—why on Earth would I cut out bread and pasta if I was never diagnosed with a wheat allergy or Celiac disease? Sugar they could understand because of the "calories"—but they didn't get why I wouldn't just switch to an artificial sweetener instead. It was very difficult and things didn't get easier for me until I began my holistic nutrition and health coaching education and found a huge tribe of like-minded people. I remember walking into my first conference and stopping dead in my tracks. Here I was in a huge room of more than 4,000 people who were all there for similar reasons and had similar stories of being judged and misunderstood for their lifestyle choices. I was elated, and I'm still a part of that community because for the first time, I was around people who didn't make me justify everything I did.

Once you decide to commit (or maybe you already have and you know what I'm talking about), you will likely run into some resistance from people close to you who just don't understand.

**My advice is this: don't explain yourself.**

You don't have to, and to be honest it won't do you or them any good. As I began to lose weight and improve my skin, people began to compliment me and tell me my skin was glowing and I looked radiant. Of course they wanted to know what I products I was using and what diet I was on that worked so well. I used to answer with a monologue that pretty much consisted of the Introduction and chapters one and two of this book! Their eyes glazed over in the first 10 seconds, but I continued talking because I felt that the more I explained myself and my choices, the more likely they would understand and give me their approval. That strategy didn't work, because the truth was that most people didn't want to hear that a lot of change and effort was involved in my transformation. They would've much rather heard that I took a magic pill, lived on grapefruits for two months, or found a miracle skincare product line.

My monologue didn't just confuse and bore people, but it began to alienate them and make them defensive. I became the health and food police. I remember one day when I was dropping my kids off at an afterschool activity. I stopped to say hello to the teacher, who was drinking an enormous, steaming hot, supersized cup of coffee from a fast food restaurant. I said hello and instead of saying hello back, she froze like a deer in headlights, her eyes opened wide, and she said "Oh no! This isn't coffee I'm drinking—I swear! It's iced tea, really!" I just laughed and said "I'm not the food police! Enjoy your coffee!" I realized that I didn't want to be the food police and I certainly didn't want people to feel defensive or uncomfortable around me. So now when people ask me what I do to keep the weight off and maintain my good skin I simply answer, "Just diet and lifestyle stuff" and they get it. Enough said.

So, while the people around you might not initially support the changes you are making or understand why you are making them, know that there are plenty of people in the exact same boat as you. There are thousands of blogs, online forums, and individual and group coaching programs or support groups available. There are also classes and workshops popping up everywhere from the smallest rural towns to the biggest cities, because health coaches are sprouting up everywhere and are excited to educate the public.

Be aware also that by adopting this new lifestyle, you are taking on the role of trendsetter! Due to the epidemics of obesity, cancer, and chronic illnesses in this country, more and more people are turning to holistic measures because they're not finding answers or cures in Western medicine. It took a very long time for our society to get to where it is today and it will take a long time for it to recover.

You're an early adapter and a trailblazer—you're a leader! While it might not seem like something you'd voluntarily sign up for, understand that your open mind and willingness to learn and experiment are very much needed. While it may not seem that people around you "get" you or your choices, they're still learning from you and eventually you'll notice that they begin to follow your example. Soon enough, the coffee drinking teacher was instead drinking huge bottles of water. I haven't gotten her on the green smoothies just yet...but she'll come around, I'm sure! So I encourage you to stand your ground and stake your claim in this movement, because not only will it change your life for the better, it'll also change the lives of those around you—whether they see it coming or not!

**Where do I begin?**

There is no "right" place to start. Some people like to dump the junk out of their kitchen cabinets and bathroom drawers immediately and start anew with a completely blank slate. Others get totally freaked out by that thought and choose to go slower by replacing products one by one as they run out of them. Food is a great starting point. The next time you go to the grocery store, look for products that have an "all natural," non-GMO, or organic alternative. You can certainly find these at farmers' markets, co-ops, and specialty health food stores, but if this isn't affordable or accessible to you, many large grocery chains now offer all natural and/ or organic store brand alternatives. Remember, the basic rule of supply and demand applies here—the more aware people become and begin to demand healthier and safer alternatives for food, personal care, and household cleaning products, the more prices will come down.

In terms of skincare and personal care products, I highly recommend you take advantage of the great work the Environmental Working Group has done with their comprehensive Skin Deep Cosmetics Database. 4 You can search for products by category, safety rating, brand name, or even look up specific ingredients. It's a great resource, and takes away a lot of the guesswork.

Many of these safer products are available in stores, and nearly all of them are available online, with helpful user reviews. You don't even have to replace your entire regimen at once...if you run out of one thing, like a cleanser before you run out of your moisturizer, just replace the cleanser for now, then replace the moisturizer once it runs out. This goes for your hair care products as well.  Eventually you'll have a full regimen of safer products.

Use the same strategy for your household products, like detergents, antibacterial wipes, and glass cleaners. There are now several brands available that contain safer ingredients for the environment and our families.

And don't forget...making your own products is always a viable, economical, and fun alternative! Don't forget to download your bonus shopping list and cleansing oil recipes at www.holisticallyhaute.com/love-your-skin-bonus-recipes.html.

**Give yourself credit where credit is due!**

Any progress made in a healthier direction is good progress, and whatever pace is comfortable for you is fine. The most important thing is that while it's good to step out of your comfort zone (and get used to doing so, by the way), you also have to be kind, gentle, and loving to yourself during every stage of the process.

There'll be setbacks and there'll be days where you just want to quit and drive directly to the ice cream shop. You might even do that, and then you'll likely feel guilty and believe that you've ruined any progress that was made. This is completely normal! We all have days where we can't or don't eat perfectly or buy a product that contains chemicals for convenience. I was visiting family once out of state and realized when I got there that I had completely forgotten my makeup—all of it. I had to go out to the store and buy new stuff and my usual brands weren't accessible. I read every label and chose as wisely as I could, wincing as I swiped my credit card to make the purchase. Setbacks will happen—it's only normal. When you have a bad diet day or miss a workout, I encourage you to tell yourself the following:

"It's OK. I love you anyway. Tomorrow will be a better day."

And then make tomorrow a better day!

**What are the biggest mistakes people make when trying to eat healthier?**

Other than little guilty pleasure indulgences and skipped workouts, there are several mistakes I've noticed that people make when they're in the beginning stages of their transition to a healthier life. Here are my top 5:

1. **Too many supplements!** Many people who are used to regularly taking prescription or OTC medications (by the way, make sure you consult with your healthcare provider about any stopping any medications you've been prescribed or adding new supplements to your regimen) really feel like taking pills is an important part of being healthy. It's just a habit, and it offers a kind of instant gratification, so they load up on supplements to substitute for medications. I'd rather see people spend their money on healthy, nutrient-dense, whole foods. Some supplements are very helpful in addition to a healthy diet, but no supplement is ever meant to be a substitute for a healthy, balanced, whole-foods based diet.

2. **Organic junk food is still junk food!** Health food newbies who are used to eating a lot of processed and packaged foods often begin their transition by switching to healthier versions of those same processed, packaged foods. If someone is going gluten-free, for example, they'll go from eating a regular prepackaged dinner to eating a gluten-free prepackaged dinner. Or if someone really loves sweets, they'll go from buying a nationally advertised brand of cookies to buying organic

cookies. A processed food is still a processed food; a junk food is still a junk food.

3.  **Recipe meltdown.** Imagine the following scenario: you get a new, healthy cookbook and are really excited to get started. You find a recipe for something that looks appealing, and you head to the grocery store to get the ingredients. The recipe calls for arame seaweed but you can't find it—all the store has is nori wraps and dulse flakes. You get discouraged and go home with a pre-packaged meal, sulking, because now you can't make the recipe since you are missing one ingredient. It's OK! Most recipes won't suffer if you leave out one single ingredient. You can also make substitutions with something similar at the store (either of those other sea vegetables would've been fine), or something you already have in your pantry or fridge (such as kale). Be creative and understand that even if you follow the recipe perfectly, it might not turn out the same as the glossy, gorgeous photograph in the book. I prefer to use recipes for inspiration and tweak them with flavors I like that I already have in my kitchen.

4.  **Information overload.** This is one of the biggest reasons people "fall off the wagon." The Internet can be a blessing or a curse, and when you begin to do searches for health-related topics you'll find very strong opinions—many of which are backed up by some kind of research—that conflict with other information. There are as many blog posts and articles saying that kale and spinach are the best foods you can put into your body as there are pointing out that raw kale contains goitrogens, which can aggravate the thyroid in large amounts, and that spinach contains oxalates, which bind to calcium and prevent absorption. Of course, most of these articles never mention that these properties pose far less risk than the chemicals in processed, food-like substances. Don't get hung up on the "research"—all research is up for interpretation these days and can be biased and taken out of context. Just enjoy your greens.

5.  **Being a converter.** Once you realize how much better you look and feel after just a couple of weeks of changing your diet and lifestyle, you'll want to scream it from the rooftops! You'll want to let everyone

know how great you feel and that they can feel that way too. You'll begin to see chronically ill people and people carrying around pill boxes full of medications and want to tell them that they don't have to live this way—that being healthy is a choice, not a sentence! Save it, trust me. Remember how crappy it felt to be at a family party reaching for a piece of cake and your mother offered you a piece of fruit instead. Remember that feeling judged sucks, and it is not your job to "fix" or "save" anyone on this planet but yourself (and your young children if you have them). Everyone is on his or her own journey, and the decision to change paths is a personal one that every person has the right to make on his or her own. It doesn't matter that you have knowledge that they don't yet have. The best you can do for them is to keep doing what you are doing and watch as it rubs off on them little by little. If they want more information, they'll ask you. If you really want to help people other than yourself and your immediate family, perhaps becoming a coach or other holistic health professional is your calling. You can only help someone who recognizes that they need help, openly asks for it, and is ready to take action.

**True health and beauty must start inside.**

What I learned in my own journey of bad skin, weight fluctuations, and self-image issues is that attempting to fix problems superficially—from the outside in—wasn't enough. I had to start inside, not just with my diet and health, but by learning to accept and truly love myself as I was. Unless I was able to love the person looking back at me in the mirror, a 200 pound woman with nasty acne at 32 years old, I knew that I'd never be happy in my life.

I don't believe that I was given this life to be miserable. I just don't believe God or the Universe or the Divine gives life for people to be miserable and do nothing with it. I believe that we're all here with a unique purpose. We're all here to serve someone or some cause. We all have special, unique gifts and talents, and we can't share them with others if we can't first honor them within ourselves.

Once I made that conscious decision and set that intention, I can't tell you how soon things started to turn around for me. The decisions that I began to make, the people that I started to attract, and the opportunities that started to open were so much more in alignment with who I really was inside. Some people might call it a miracle, or the Law of Attraction, or even magic—but that would imply that it all happened by chance. I do believe in the universal Law of Attraction, but in order for that to work, one must first take clear and consistent action.

While healing a skin condition and losing weight might seem like physical acts, we have to remember that every aspect of our whole self is interconnected: the mind, body, and spirit. Ayurveda teaches that all consciousness and existence begins with the soul—the spirit.

My favorite self-love author and teacher, Christine Arylo, taught me that,

*"Self-love is a spiritual journey - one that affects our minds, our bodies, and every experience in our lives. Self-love is not something that you achieve one day so you can move on to the next spiritual growth milestone, self-love is a daily choice. In every moment of every day, do you choose love instead of fear, judgment, criticism, hate, etc.? When you are on the path of self-love, your ability to choose love for yourself increases, and so does your ability to give love to others.*

### What is self-love, and how do you know if you are loving yourself well?

*There are ten branches of self-love including self-acceptance, self-esteem, self-care, self-compassion - all related but all distinct. Self- acceptance, for example, is truly loving who you are for exactly who you are; all of it . The brilliant parts of you that are easy to love, and the 'imperfections' that are harder to love. Your job as your own best friend is to cultivate deep self-acceptance by loving every single part of you. To be a lover not a hater of every piece of you.*

*All healing stems from love. Those of us who have physical marks or scars on our bodies may find it difficult to love the parts of our bodies that don't match the external standard for beauty, but there is another choice when you use the self-love power of self-acceptance. If you were to look at that part of your body with the same eyes you would as a child who was born with a physical 'imperfection' or a best friend who had a change in their body, what would you say to to yourself about this body part? Not in a way to gloss over the body part, but to really be with it and find the beauty within it, to find the teaching and the message it had for you? What could you learn about yourself? This inquiry is the road to true self-acceptance, which ultimately frees you to be who you are, without apology, without shame. All scars and blemishes have the power to heal you from the inside out. Your job is to choose to look at those scars and blemishes with new eyes, the eyes of a best friend."*

You're a unique, talented, beautiful being that was born from love. Even if the topics of self-image, acceptance, and love are uncomfortable for you, just know that the more love you give, the more you'll receive, and the faster you'll heal from whatever it is that ails you. While your natural tendency might be to give that love away to other people, remember that you need and deserve love too—so start with you. Don't worry, there is never a shortage of love. Once you give some to yourself, there'll be plenty more to give to others, and you'll notice that the more you love yourself the more love you will begin to receive from others.

Self-love is the catalyst that'll make the rest of your journey fall in line. You'll begin to realize that healthy choices are the ONLY choices, because you are worthy of nothing but the best. Negative words and actions from others will begin to seem irrelevant, because you'll no longer seek external approval and validation. It starts with you, and ultimately, ends with you; everything in between is all about you even when others are involved. This doesn't make you selfish, vain, or narcissistic—it makes you appreciative of the beautiful life that you were given.

You know how wonderful it feels when you give a gift to someone and their eyes just light up as they say, "Thank you, thank you! I love it!" Your skin, your health, your body, your emotions, your spirit, and your life are the greatest gifts you can receive. Choose to love and honor them!

# Glossary

**Acid mantle**—the matrix of different proteins, cells, sebum, sweat, and various other cells, fluids, and lipids that holds the outermost layers of the skin together.

**Adipose tissue:** Layer of fat located below the dermis that gives contour and shape to the body. It provides a protective cushion for the skeleton and vital organs underneath. This fat layer, like the dermis above it, thins with age. Also referred to as, "subcutaneous fat layer" or "subcutis".

**Angel dusting:** A loophole that allows manufacturers to advertise expensive ingredients on product labels, packaging, and marketing materials as long as the product contains a minimum percentage of that ingredient. This percentage is often too low for the ingredient to actually provide any **benefit.**

**Antioxidant:** "A substance, such as vitamin C, vitamin E, or beta carotene that counteracts the damaging effects of oxidation from free radicals in a living organism"[22].

**Ayurveda:** A holistic practice of healing the mind, body, and spirit that originated in India more than 5,000 years ago.

**Basal layer:** The deepest layer of the epidermis, which rests on the dermis and is where melanocytes are located.

**Candida albicans:** A particularly resistant strain of yeast that naturally occurs in various parts of the body which feeds on decomposing tissue, sugars, and other substances in the body. Its main job in the body is to decompose tissue postmortem. When it overgrows, it outnumbers healthy strains of bacteria and microflora in the body causing many symptoms such as skin conditions and other inflammatory conditions of the body.

**Chemical Exfoliation:** Also sometimes referred to as chemical peeling. It is performed by topically applying enzymes, or alpha or beta hydroxy acids to the epidermis with the intention of wounding certain layers of the skin, thus causing inflammation. The idea behind this is that the wound created will send a message to the brain to produce new collagen and speed up the cell turnover rate.

**Collagen:** A very strong and pliable protein produced in the dermis by fibroblasts that supports the bones, joints, and connective tissues including the skin. Collagen makes up approximately 70% of the dermis. Its rate of production is affected by the aging process as well as diet, lifestyle, and environmental factors.

**Corneocytes:** "Dead", or flattened, keratinocytes that comprise the outermost layer of the epidermis and are shed regularly.

**Cortisol:** Also known as the "fight or flight hormone", or "the stress hormone". When cortisol is released, it takes over the parts of the brain that are normally regulated by hormones that keep us happy, even-tempered, and thinking clearly. Instead, the response is similar to that of adrenaline: thoughts are urgent, hyper, sometimes manic.

**Dermatitis**—see "Eczema"

**Dermatology:** A branch of conventional Western medicine that specializes in the diagnosis and treatment of diseases of the skin.

**Dermis:** The deeper layers of the skin which house blood vessels, nerve endings, fibroblasts, hair follicles containing sebaceous and sudoriferous glands, and other tissue. The dermis is located between the epidermis and the adipose tissue.

**Detoxification:** Also referred to as "internal cleansing"— is the process of removing built up toxins from the body.

**Eczema:** An inflammatory skin condition with symptoms such as dry, scaly patches—areas that are crusty, flaky, and thick, which can sometimes ooze and are often red and very itchy.

**Elastin:** A protein produced in the dermis by fibroblasts similar to collagen that provides strength and elasticity to the skin and other connective tissues. This protein degrades due to aging, poor diet and lifestyle factors, and environmental factors.

**Elastosis:** Loss of elasticity in the skin that occurs when fibroblasts no longer produce elastin, mostly due to damage from overexposure over time to the sun's UV radiation.

**Emollient:** A substance that lies on the surface of the skin providing nourishment, lubrication, enhancing softness and pliability, and locking in hydration.

**Enzyme:** Chemicals that, when activated by certain catalysts, break up or digest protein fibers.

**Epidermis:** The outermost layer of the skin which serves as protection and continuously sheds itself and is replaced by new cells.

**Essential fatty acid (EFA):** A type of fat that the body needs but does not produce enough of on its own. These fats, such as alpha linolenic acid (ALA) and docosahexaenoic acid (DHA) are vital for proper growth and function of nearly every cell in the body. The correct balance of EFAs provides protection and lubrication to the cell membranes and also has been shown to reduce inflammation.

**Essential oil:** Natural aromatic compounds found in the seeds, bark, stems, roots, flowers, and other parts of plants. In addition to giving plants their distinctive smells, essential oils provide plants with protection against predators and disease and play a role in plant pollination. Essential oils have also been used throughout history in many cultures for their medicinal and therapeutic benefits.[45]

**Exfoliation:** The naturally occurring shedding of accumulated dead skin cells from the epidermis. This process is also done manually, electronically, mechanically, and chemically with certain skincare products and treatments.

**Fibroblasts:** Cells located in the dermis responsible for producing collagen and elastin

**Free radicals:** Highly unstable, unpaired (single) electrons. When anything happens to energize or "excite" these single electrons, they steal an electron from a healthy pair in order to stabilize themselves, thus breaking up that pair and leaving that electron single and unstable. This process causes a chain reaction and may lead to DNA or cellular mutation.

**Ghee:** Butter that has been clarified by removing the casein to make it more digestible.

**Gluten:** A protein found in wheat, barley, corn, and other whole grains and seeds. It is also frequently added to processed foods in order to meet protein requirements.

**Histology:** A branch of anatomy that deals with the minute structure of animal and plant tissues as discernible with the microscope.[44]

**Holistic:** Also referred to as "wholistic" — the philosophy and practice of healing that has to do with constantly keeping the whole body at the highest level of total wellness. It goes back to the universal natural law that states that a whole is made up of the sum of all of its parts, and that the parts cannot function properly if the whole is not functioning properly. Conversely, if there is a problem with one of the parts, the entire whole is affected.

**Holistic skincare:** Using nutrition and healthy lifestyle choices in addition to high quality, natural skincare products to nourish and protect the skin from the inside out and outside in.

**Humectant:** A substance that ability to draw, retain, and bind water.

**Hyaluronic acid (HA):** A protein produced in the dermis that is abundant in our skin and bodies at birth, and degrades as we age and with overexposure to the sun's radiation. It has strong humectant properties and can hold 1,000 times its own molecular weight in water. It is a component of the skin's natural moisturizing factor, and provides lubrication to other cells and tissues in the body. HA is also crucial to reducing inflammation and aiding the body's wound healing process.

**Hyperpigmentation:** Dark spots or discolorations on the skin that form when a melanocyte produces excess melanin pigment due to damage or mutation from inflammation, oxidation, or trauma.

**Keratinocytes:** The predominant cells located throughout the epidermis that produce keratin—a protein found in the skin, hair, and nails. Keratinocytes originate in the basal layer and travel through the different layers of the epidermis, where they flatten and eventually "die; they are shed as corneocytes.

**Keratosis pilaris:** "Chicken skin" or goosebump-like textured skin often found on the knees, thighs, buttocks, forearms, elbows, upper arms, and sometimes shoulders. This condition may indicate Vitamin A deficiency or gluten intolerance.

**Light emitting diode (LED) therapy:** Topically delivers a combination of visible light (typically red or blue light which each have different therapeutic properties) and healing infrared rays with the intention of improving the appearance and health of the skin by encouraging production of new collagen and elastin.

**Melanocytes:** Cells found in the basal layer of the epidermis that produce the body's melanin pigment

**Melasma:** A specific type of hyperpigmentation, which almost always appears on the face with a specific and symmetrical mask-like pattern, often covering the forehead, cheeks, chin, jawline, and upper lip. The severity of the amount of pigment varies based on how much melanin pigment the person naturally has. Those with lighter complexions are affected less, while those with more pigmented complexions are more likely to develop this condition. This condition is often called "mask of pregnancy", although it may develop from other causes such as inflammation and free radical damage.

**Microcurrent:** An electrotherapy treatment that releases a very small amount of alternating current in a concentrated area and actually retrains the facial muscles to firm up instead of sag.

**Microdermabrasion:** An electronic form of mechanical exfoliation that uses micro-crystals or crushed diamonds to essentially "sand" the surface of the skin. It also utilizes strong suction, which helps remove embedded dead cells and debris.

**Microneedling:** A technique that uses a small, handheld wheel covered in tiny acupuncture needles of different lengths. This device is rolled onto the skin to "open up" the pores. It also superficially wounds the skin which, in theory, causes the dermis to produce more collagen and elastin to plump, smooth, and firm up the skin. It is also used to improve the penetration of active skin care ingredients.

**Naturopathic doctor:** A holistic physician who specializes in treating the whole person, identifying causes rather than treating symptoms, preventing illness, educating and consulting with patients, and using herbs and other natural compounds to assist the body's effort to heal itself.

**Nutriceutical:** A food or naturally occurring food supplement thought to have a beneficial effect on human health.[46] The FDA does not regulate dietary supplements or recognize this as a valid term—the term is more used for marketing purposes and does not determine a product's efficacy.

**Occlusive:** A substance that sits on the surface of the skin and does not allow the passage of air or moisture, often resulting in suffocated skin.

**Oxidation:** the chemical reaction that occurs when oxygen is added to a substance. This causes a loss of electrons, which leads to a change in the chemical properties of the substance, transforming it into something different from its original form.

**Pasteurization:** The process of heating substances (often food products) to extremely high temperatures to kill bacteria, fungi, or viruses.

**Probiotics:** Beneficial strains of bacteria, yeasts, and other microflora that live primarily in the gastrointestinal tract, aiding digestion and detoxification. Probiotics boost the body's immune system by keeping pathogen levels under control.

**Psoriasis:** An autoimmune disease that not only manifests as flare-ups of red, scaly lesions on the skin, but also as psoriatic arthritis. Flare-ups can be prevented and treated holistically and medically.

**Rosacea:** A persistent, chronic disorder of the skin and sometimes the eyes that is characterized by an inflammatory redness usually on the nose and cheeks but sometimes elsewhere; swelling, small and visible dilated or distended ("broken") capillaries, bumps and acne pustules, irritated and watery eyes, and in severe cases, areas of thickened skin which could lead to disfigurement.

**Sebaceous glands:** Glands located in the root of the hair follicles in the dermis responsible for secreting sebum.

**Seborrhea:** A skin disorder characterized by over-productive sebaceous glands and an overabundance of sebum.

**Sebum:** Oily, wax-like substance secreted by the sebaceous glands which provides protection and lubrication to the skin.

**Serum:** A highly concentrated skincare product containing higher amounts of therapeutic ingredients specially formulated to penetrate into the deeper layers of the skin.

**Skin Trigger Trifecta:** The three foods/substances—gluten, dairy, and refined sugar—that are known to trigger skin conditions such as acne, eczema, rosacea, psoriasis, keratosis pilaris, melasma, and seborrhea.

**Stevia:** A naturally sweet herb native to South America that is commonly used as an alternative to sugar and artificial sweeteners. Stevia does not contain sugar and does not produce a glycemic reaction.

**Stratum germanitivum**—see "Basal layer"

**Subcutaneous fat** –see"Adipose"

**Sudoriferous glands:** Glands located within the hair follicles in the dermis that excrete sweat.

**Trans-epidermal Water Loss (TEWL):** Loss of water from the body via evaporation through the skin.

**Trans-fat or trans-fatty acid:** A highly industrial process where artificial fats are made by adding hydrogen to oils and then rearranging them on a molecular level. During this process, these oils are hardened to more closely resemble butter and make them stable enough to prevent rancidity and keep them intact at high temperatures.

**Vasodilation:** When capillaries and other blood vessels dilate in an effort to circulate more blood and nutrients to a specific part of the body. This often results in visibly distended capillaries on the skin. After repeated occurrences, the vessels may dilate permanently.

# References

1. Environmental Working Group: The Power of Information. http://www. ewg.org/. Accessed July 14, 2013.

2. The Campaign for Safe Cosmetics. http://safecosmetics.org/. Accessed July 14, 2013.

3. Pontillo R. Ingredient spotlight: Vitamin A in skincare. Holistically Haute™ website. http://www.holisticallyhaute.com/2011/08/ ingredient-spotlight-vitamin-a-in-skin-care.html. August 20, 2011. Accessed July 14, 2013.

4. EWG's Skin Deep® Cosmetics Database page. Environmental Working Group website. http://www.ewg.org/skindeep/. Accessed July 14, 2013.

5. Pontillo R. Lifestyle upgrade! 8 tips to improve your daily routine. Holistically Haute™ website. http://www.holisticallyhaute. com/2012/08/lifestyle-upgrade-8-easy-tips-to-improve-your-daily- routine.html. August 27, 2012. Accessed July 14, 2013.

6. Pontillo R. "Chin and neck massage at home" video. Holistically Haute™ YouTube channel. http://www.youtube.com/watch?v=FgCznEXagNQ. December 14, 2011. Accessed July 14, 2013.

7. Pontillo R. What do your eyes reveal about your health? Holistically Haute™ website. http://www.holisticallyhaute.com/2011/08/what-do- your-eyes-reveal-about-your-health.html. August 10, 2011. Accessed July 14, 2013.

8. Francis R and Cotton K. Never Be Sick Again: Health is a Choice, Learn How to Choose it. Deerfield Beach, FL: Health Communications, Inc. 2002.

9. What are we eating? Label GMOs.org website. http://www.labelgmos.

org/the_science_genetically_modified_foods_gmo. Accessed July 14, 2013.

10. Shaw J. Gravid bovines modern milk. Harvard Magazine. 2007; May-June. http://www.labelgmos.org/the_science_genetically_modified_foods_gmo. Accessed July 14, 2013.

11. Dr. Linda T. Nelson, PhD, RND. M'lis website. http://www.mlis.com/dr-linda-t-nelson-n-d-ph-d-founder-and-ceo-1000284. Accessed July 14, 2013.

12. Nelson L. Living Symptom Free: Fibromyalgia & Candida: A Comprehensive Resource Written to Help You Live Symptom Free from Degenerative Disease within Six months. 3rd Edition. Salt Lake City, UT: Beneficial International. 2002: 96.

13. Pontillo R. The detox toolbox: dry brushing. Holistically Haute™ website. http://www.holisticallyhaute.com/2011/06/the-detox-toolbox-dry-brushing.html. June 3, 2011. Accessed July 14, 2013.

14. Mosher HH. Simultaneous study of constituents of urine and perspiration. J Biol Chem. 1933, 99:781-790. http://www.jbc.org/content/99/3/781.full.pdf+html. Accessed July 14, 2013.

15. Pollan M. In Defense of Food: An Eater's Manifesto: New York, NY: The Penguin Press; 2008

16. Santa Maria C. The real definition of insanity. The Huffington Post website. http://www.huffingtonpost.com/2011/12/20/insanity-definition_n_1159927.html. December 20, 2011. Accessed July 14, 2013.

17. Pontillo R. What's the most addictive drug? The answer might surprise you. Holistically Haute™ website. http://www.holisticallyhaute.com/2012/03/whats-the-most-addictive-drug-the-answer-may-surprise-you.html. March 21, 2012. Accessed July 14, 2013.

18. Pontillo R. Don't worry about the plants...water yourself! Holistically Haute™ website. http://www.holisticallyhaute.com/2011/01/dont-

worry-about-the-plants-water-yourself.html. January 6, 2011. Accessed July 14, 2013.

19. Mercola J. The forbidden food you should never stop eating. Mercola.com website. http://articles.mercola.com/sites/articles/ archive/2011/09/01/enjoy-saturated-fats-theyre-good-for-you.aspx. September 1, 2011. Accessed July 14, 2013.

20. Weston A. Price Foundation®. http://www.westonaprice.org/. Accessed July 14, 2013.

21. Pontillo R. Fighting off free radicals: Antioxidants. Holistically Haute™ website. http://www.holisticallyhaute.com/2011/03/fighting-off-free-radicals-antioxidants.html. March 2, 2011. Accessed July 14, 2013.

22. Antioxidant. Dictionary.com website. http://dictionary.reference.com/ browse/antioxidant. Accessed July 14, 2013.

23. Pontillo R. What are these free radicals I keep hearing about? Holistically Haute™ website. http://www.holisticallyhaute. com/2011/01/what-are-these-free-radicals-i-keep-hearing-about.html. January 23, 2011. Accessed July 14, 2013.

24. Pontillo R. Recipe: Citrus arugula salad with red quinoa and mixed seeds. Holistically Haute™ website. http://www.holisticallyhaute. com/2012/09/recipe-citrus-arugula-salad-with-red-quinoa-and-mixed-seeds.html. September 25, 2012. Accessed July 14, 2013.

25. Health Coach Starter Guide. The Institute for Integrative Nutrition® website. http://www.integrativenutrition.com/Health-Coach-Starter-Guide?erefer=0015000000alkyZAAS. Accessed July 14, 2013.

26. EWG's Shopper's Guide to Pesticides in Produce™ The Environmental Working Group website. http://www.ewg.org/foodnews/. Accessed July 14, 2013.

27. Pontillo R. Addicted to tanning? Technorati™ website. http:// technorati.com/lifestyle/article/addicted-to-tanning/. June 11, 2011. Accessed July 14, 2013.

28. Dermatology: There's no safe tan. Massachusetts General Hospital website. http://www.massgeneral.org/dermatology/news/newsarticle. aspx?id=2210. May 14, 2010. Accessed July 14, 2013.

29. Pontillo R. Stress less: look and feel your best. Holistically Haute™ website. http://www.holisticallyhaute.com/2011/01/stress-less-look-and-feel-your-best.html. January 10, 2011. Accessed July 14, 2013.

30. Slominski A. A nervous breakdown in the skin: stress and the epidermal barrier. J Clin Invest. 2007 November 1; 117(11): 3166–3169. http://www.ncbi.nlm.nih.gov/pmc/articles/PMC2045620/. Accessed July 14, 2013.

31. Kresser C. The gut-skin connection: how altered gut function affects the skin. Chris Kresser L. Ac: Medicine for the 21st Century website. http://chriskresser.com/the-gut-skin-connection-how-altered-gut-function-affects-the-skin. October 19, 2012. Accessed July 14, 2013.

32. Pontillo R. How smoking affects your skin. Holistically Haute™ website. http://www.holisticallyhaute.com/2011/03/how-smoking-affects-your-skin.html. March 29, 2011. Accessed July 14, 2013.

33. The effects of smoking on the skin (the full article). StopSmokingToday. com website. http://www.stopsmokingtoday.com/dyn/126/The-Effects-of-Smoking-on-the-Skin.html. Accessed July 14, 2013.

34. Pontillo R. Air pollution: one of the greatest causes of skin problems. Holistically Haute™ website. http://www.holisticallyhaute. com/2011/04/air-pollution-one-of-the-greatest-causes-of-skin-problems.html. April 14, 2011. Accessed July 14, 2013.

35. Keefer A. Air pollution effects on skin. Livestrong.com: The Unlimited Potential of You website. http://www.livestrong.com/article/145802-air-pollution-effects-on-skin/. June 11, 2010. Accessed July 14, 2013.

36. Pontillo R. Why synthetic fragrances stink. Blogcritics: The Critical Lens on Today's Culture & Entertainment website. http://blogcritics.org/why-synthetic-fragrances-stink/. May 5, 2011. Accessed July 14, 2013.

37. Guide to less toxic products. Enviromental Health Association of Nova Scotia website. http://www.lesstoxicguide.ca/index.asp?fetch=usage. Accessed July 14, 2013.

38. Pontillo R. What's the big deal about parabens? Holistically Haute™ website. http://www.holisticallyhaute.com/2011/03/what-is-the-big-deal-about-parabens.html. March 8, 2011. Accessed July 14, 2013.

39. Darbre, P D, Aljarrah, A, Miller, WR, Coldham, NG, Sauer, MJ, and Pope, GS. (2004), Concentrations of parabens in human breast tumours. J. Appl. Toxicol., 24: 5–13. doi: 10.1002/jat.958 Accessed July 14, 2013.

40. Meeker JD, Yang T, Ye X, Calafat AM, and Hauser R. Urinary concentrations of parabens and serum hormone levels, semen quality parameters, and sperm DNA damage. Environ Health Perspect. 2011 February; 119(2): 252–257. Published online 2010 September 28. doi: 10.1289/ehp.1002238. Accessed July 14, 2013.

41. Darbre PD, Harvey PW. Paraben esters: review of recent studies of endocrine toxicity, absorption, esterase and human exposure, and discussion of potential human health risks. J Appl Toxicol. 2008 Jul;28(5):561-78. doi: 10.1002/jat.1358. Accessed July 14, 2013.

42. Trow C, Trow R. The truth about parabens. Skin Inc. http://www.skininc.com/skinscience/ingredients/97476464.html?page=1. June 30, 2010. Accessed July 14, 2013.

43. AromaTools. Modern Essentials: A Contemporary Guide to the Therapeutic Use of Essential Oils, 3rd edition. Spanish Fork, UT: Abundant Health, LLC; 2012.

44. Definition of "histology". Merriam Webster website. http://www.merriam-webster.com/medical/histology. Accessed July 14, 2013.

45. What is an essential oil? The Holistically Haute™ dōTERRA® website, IPC #327471. http://www.mydoterra.com/holisticallyhaute/essentialDefinition.html. Accessed July 14, 2013.

46. Nutriceutical. The Free Dictionary by Farlex website. http://medical-dictionary.thefreedictionary.com/nutriceutical. Accessed July 14, 2013.

# About the Author

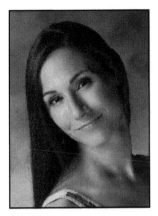

Rachael Pontillo is an author, speaker, and AADP certified Holistic Health and Image Coach with more than 15 years of experience in the beauty and healthcare industries. Following her own challenges with acne and weight, she has helped many women overcome skin conditions and self image issues in her private coaching practice.

She is the founder and publisher of the popular blog, Holistically Haute™, at www.holisticallyhaute.com, and her work has been featured in top aesthetics trade journals and health and wellness publications and websites around the world.

Rachael received her holistic nutrition and coaching education and certification from the Institute for Integrative Nutrition®; her aesthetics education from The Vision Academy, a Paul Mitchell partner school; and her Bachelor of Science degree from Philadelphia University. She has received continuing education from the Arizona Center for Integrative Medicine and the International Dermal Institute on the subjects of health, detoxification, Ayurveda, Traditional Chinese Medicine, and advanced aesthetics. Rachael is also a level II Reiki practitioner.

Rachael is a recipient of the Institute for Integrative Nutrition's prestigious Health Leadership Award, and is a featured skincare expert and ambassador for the holistic skincare supplement company, NeoCell™.

Made in the USA
San Bernardino, CA
10 June 2020

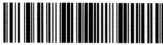